Positive Therapy

T0092770

The applications of positive psychology are different from traditional interventions in therapy in that they are focused on building strength, resilience and well-being rather than being restricted to simply treating disorder. Since the publication of the first edition of *Positive Therapy*, there is now a comprehensive body of applied positive psychology research to which practitioners may turn in order to inform their own practice, and that sees its purpose as the facilitation of human flourishing and optimal functioning.

However, much of this research and its implications are only now becoming more widely understood in counselling and psychotherapy. This new edition of *Positive Therapy* shows how the latest thinking in positive psychology can be applied to psychotherapeutic practice, and specifically to person-centred therapy. Making the links between positive psychology and psychotherapy explicit, Stephen Joseph describes the new tools that practitioners can draw upon to help and facilitate positive functioning in their clients. New material includes:

- An update of the latest positive psychology research
- A new preface, explaining how positive psychology principles can now be applied to therapeutic practice
- Focus on positive psychology measurement tools

Positive Therapy will be essential reading for all psychotherapists, counsellors, social workers, coaches, psychologists and trainees interested in exploring how they engage with clients, and the implications of this engagement in practice.

Stephen Joseph is a professor in the School of Education at the University of Nottingham where he is convenor for the counselling and psychotherapy group. He is a registered counselling psychologist. Stephen has published widely on positive psychology, psychological trauma and therapy.

"This book is a milestone. It takes the humanistic approach to the 21st century and stresses its potential to become a metatheory. Sharp, and yet deeply insightful, this book integrates academic kudos with the authentic heart and soul of a person centred therapist. Stephen has managed to revisit the language and convey the core of the approach in a fresh and approachable to all manner."

– Zoë Chouliara, Reader in Person Centred Care,
Edinburgh Napier University, Practitioner Counselling
Psychologist & Person Centred Psychotherapist/Counsellor

"Stephen Joseph takes us on a captivating journey through the latest developments in Positive Psychology and Person-Centred Theory and Practice, eloquently making the case for an integration of these two traditions based upon a meta-theoretical understanding that is underpinned by empirical findings from positive psychology and grounded in the person-centred theoretical account of the *actualising tendency*. The actualising tendency, the bedrock of the person-centred approach, represents the view that all humans have an inherent tendency to be self-determining agents of their own directions in life and that, consequently, clients in therapy should always be regarded as *their own best experts*. With potentially profound implications for psychotherapeutic practice, this book is a must read for therapists and psychologists alike and indeed for anyone curious to learn more about an empirically supported and refreshingly alternative paradigm to the dominant medical model of psychological distress."

– Tom Patterson, Clinical Psychologist and
Senior Lecturer in Clinical Psychology,
Coventry University, UK

"This book is an extremely valuable contribution to the fields of positive psychology and person-centered psychotherapy, exploring the synergy between the two approaches, and the way of combining them in clinical practice. The book is filled with practical suggestions, scientific studies and the rich experiences of the author as a skilfull practitioner. Specifically, this new edition presents what person-centred therapists have to gain from positive psychology and on the other hand how positive psychologist can benefit from it in order to reach a deeper appreciation of the richness of person-centered approach and integrate these ideas into their practice. A wonderful book, engaging, relevant and comprehensive, completed with new material and new sections on person-activity fit and theoretically consistent measurement."

– Antonia Csillik, Ph.D., Senior Lecturer
in clinical psychology, University of Paris
Ouest Nanterre, France, Vice-President of
the French speaking Positive Psychology Association,
member of the Motivational Interviewing
Network of Trainers, MINT

Positive Therapy

Building bridges between
positive psychology and
person-centred therapy

Second edition

Stephen Joseph

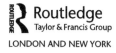

Routledge
Taylor & Francis Group

LONDON AND NEW YORK

Second edition published 2015
by Routledge
27 Church Road, Hove, East Sussex, BN3 2FA

and by Routledge
711 Third Avenue, New York, NY 10017

Routledge is an imprint of the Taylor & Francis Group, an informa business

British Library Cataloguing in Publication Data
A catalogue record for this book is available from the British Library

First edition published by Routledge in 2006.

Library of Congress Cataloging-in-Publication Data
Joseph, Stephen (College teacher)
[Positive therapy]
Positive psychology : building bridges between positive psychology and
person-centred therapy / Stephen Joseph. — Second Edition.
pages cm
Revised edition of the author's Positive therapy, 2006.
1. Positive psychology. 2. Psychotherapy. I. Title.
BF204.6.J67 2015
158'.9—dc23
2014044704

ISBN: 978-0-415-72341-1 (hbk)
ISBN: 978-0-415-72342-8 (pbk)
ISBN: 978-1-315-74290-8 (ebk)

Typeset in Times New Roman
by Swales & Willis Ltd, Exeter, Devon, UK

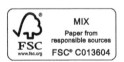

Contents

Figures and tables

Preface

The first edition of this book was published in 2006. At that time many therapists were becoming interested in how the new ideas of positive psychology could be applied to psychotherapy. Used to thinking only in terms of symptom reduction, they were now asking how they could facilitate positive functioning in their clients. Unbeknownst to many of those asking this question, several decades earlier the humanistic psychologist Carl Rogers had already tackled this very question. His approach to therapy was based on the meta-theoretical assumption that people have an inherent tendency towards growth, development and becoming fully functioning. But these do not happen automatically. For people to actualize their inherent optimal nature they require the right social environment. Without the right social environment the inherent tendency towards growth can become thwarted and usurped, leading instead to psychological distress and dysfunction. For Rogers, fully functioning meant more than simply the absence of distress and dysfunction. It implied, for example, that a person was self-directed, autonomous and open to experience. In this way, Rogers' approach was a positive psychology before the term was invented. The first edition of this book set out to build bridges between positive psychology and the humanistic person-centred therapy of Carl Rogers.

Positive therapy, as I mean it, is essentially a person-centred approach but one that embraces the theory and research of positive psychology. Since the first edition, the idea of positive therapy has attracted a great deal of attention. The invitation to revise the book has given me the opportunity to update it with the new developments in theory and research of the last decade and to refine my thinking on positive therapy.

Specifically, this new edition allows me to present more clearly what person-centred therapists have to gain from positive psychology. Since the first edition, there has been a growing awareness among person-centred therapists of positive psychology. But as yet there is not the full recognition of what it can offer them. Notably there are two main ways in which person-centred therapists can benefit from positive psychology. First, there is theory and research in positive psychology that supports person-centred therapy. Second, there are measurement tools developed by positive psychologists that are theoretically consistent with person-centred therapy that can complement and replace the traditional symptom-focused measures. In my view the theory and research of positive psychology enhances and strengthens person-centred therapy. Some may find what I have to say controversial but I hope that most will understand what I have written as encouraging of the development of the person-centred approach. I endeavour to be person-centred in my own approach to therapy. For me it is an ethical stance of respect for the self-determination of others, and nothing I say in this book is intended to contravene that position. If at times it seems that I do then I would ask the reader to consider it clumsiness in my expression rather than in my intent.

On the other side of the fence, positive psychologists have also begun to engage with ideas once associated with the person-centred approach such as the meta-theory of the tendency towards actualization and the important role of human rela-tionships in well-being. I hope that positive psychologists who are less familiar with the person-centred approach will come away from this book with a deeper appreciation of the depth and richness of person-centred approach and be inspired to integrate these ideas into their own practice.

One theme that runs throughout the book is the notion of non-directive practice. Non-directivity is a much misunderstood concept. It does not mean unstructured, sloppy or passive but refers to actively following the direction of the client, closely, carefully and creatively. As we come to understand this concept more closely I hope to show how practitioners can work within this framework in spontaneous and flexible ways that are responsive to the moment-by-moment needs of their clients.

I also say goodbye in this edition to Alex Linley who helped me author the first edition. I wish him well in his new endeavours. As with the previous edition, the vision for positive therapy I present in this book is a work in progress, as the ideas are constantly evolving, but this time it is a single authored vision for positive therapy. One of the main changes I have made to the book is the subtitle: 'Build-ing bridges between positive psychology and person-centred psychotherapy'. This title better reflects what the book is about and how it is a two-way dialogue that I am encouraging between positive psychology and person-centred therapy. I have also added new material throughout the book, especially new sections on person-activity fit and theoretically consistent measurement.

There are other textbooks that provide a more comprehensive discussion of either the person-centred approach or positive psychology, and readers will find plenty of references to other sources throughout, but what is unique about this book is that it seeks to explore the synergy between the two disciplines, and looks to a future where there is no longer a need for bridge building. My aim is that person-centred therapy be seen not only in its historical context as a form of humanistic therapy but that it becomes recognized more widely as an example of positive psychology in practice, and a much needed one in contemporary society where the self-determination of individuals seems under increasing threat.

This book is intended for all those interested in helping people flourish. I hope all those interested in the applications of positive psychology and the person-centred approach will find this book helpful. Specifically, the book is written with graduate students in positive psychology interested in psychotherapy, and trainees in person-centred therapy curious about positive psychology, in mind. I hope you enjoy this book and find things in it that inspire you in your learning and practice.

Stephen Joseph
July, 2014

Acknowledgements

Thanks to Carol Kauffman, Tom Patterson and Richard Worsley for their encouragement, helpful advice and suggestions during the first edition, Zoe Chouliara, Mick Cooper, Antonia Csillik, Kate Hefferon, Chiara Ruini and David Murphy for their helpful discussions during the writing of this second edition. Thanks to Joanne Forshaw at Routledge for her enthusiasm for the project and for her invitation to do a second edition.

Chapter 1

Introduction

Positive therapy is about helping people become more fully functioning. Put another way, if the traditional goal of therapy is to help the patient move from −5 to 0 the positive therapist is interested in how to help them move from −5 to +5. Changing the terms of therapy in this way has significant implications. It alters how we think about what we are doing. We begin to have different conversations with our clients. We listen to our clients in new ways. We begin to think about the nature of their suffering differently. In this chapter I will set the scene for the book by very briefly introducing positive psychology, the humanistic approach of Carl Rogers and the idea of positive therapy.

Positive psychology

Most readers will have heard the term positive psychology and may already know something about it, but may not appreciate that it is a serious branch of applied psychology with a growing tradition of scholarly research behind it. Positive psychology was an idea that developed at the turn of the new century when it was formally launched by Martin Seligman in his Presidential Address to the American Psychological Association (APA) in 1998. Seligman's argument was that for too long psychologists had looked only at the negative and destructive side of human experience. Surely it was as important, perhaps even more so, to understand what is positive and constructive. Thus there followed scholars and practitioners interested in finding out about human flourishing, happiness and how people can achieve the best in themselves.

Since these beginnings positive psychology has developed into an area of sophisticated scholarship that seeks to understand and promote the study of what is good about life. Attention has also focused on how research findings may be applied in practical settings. Areas of application span clinical, educational, forensic, health and organizational domains. The applications of positive psychology are different from traditional interventions in that they are focused on building strengths, well-being and resilience, rather than simply treating disorder and dysfunction. In this sense, it might be said that whereas traditional psychology was concerned with −5 to 0 the new positive psychology was concerned with 0 to +5.

The ideas of positive psychology are now also entering the consciousness of the therapeutic counselling and psychotherapy community. For many in therapeutic counselling and psychotherapy these are brand new ideas that challenge them to rethink their approach to therapy. For others, these ideas sound familiar. Indeed, as I will go on to show, it is now recognized that humanistic psychology was a forerunner of positive psychology (Taylor, 2001; Resnick, Warmoth, & Serlin, 2001; Robbins, 2015). One of the pioneers of humanistic psychology and humanistic therapy was Carl Rogers. It is to him and his work that we now turn.

The humanistic psychology of Carl Rogers

Rogers was originally a psychologist by training. In 1947 he served as the President of the American Psychological Association, the position held by Seligman 50 years later when he founded the positive psychology movement. Rogers had many scholarly achievements in his life. One of his earliest achievements was to pioneer psychotherapy research. Using the cutting edge technology of the 1940s, Rogers was the first psychologist to use recordings of therapeutic sessions for research. By recording his interviews on 78 rpm records, which were then transcribed, and publishing the verbatim transcripts for research, Rogers and his colleagues put the spotlight on what actually went on during therapy. It is hard to imagine from the perspective of today when we take such research for granted just how radical it was to subject the intricacies and secrets of the psychotherapy session to rigorous scientific examination. A complete issue of the *Journal of Consulting Psychology* was devoted to the research in 1948 (see Farber, Brink, & Raskin, 1996). It was through his observations of therapy and subsequent research that Rogers developed his own approach to practice which was based on the notion that clients have the solutions to their difficulties within themselves. Nowadays this idea is taken for granted in many ways but back then to question the idea of the therapist as expert over the other person in terms of knowing what hurts and what is needed was truly a radical idea.

In 1942 Rogers published his first major work entitled *Counseling and Psychotherapy: Newer concepts in practice*, in which he presented his approach which he referred to as *non-directive therapy*. He described it as non-directive therapy because it was the therapist's task to follow the client's lead, thus challenging the then dominant therapist-directed approaches of psychoanalysis and behaviourism. Rather than the therapist directing the course of therapy by using interpretative methods or reinforcement schedules to derive solutions for the patient, Rogers turned the notion of the therapist as the expert upside down. His focus was on reflection of feelings in such a way as to shift the direction of sessions so that the therapist followed the client, helping them to uncover their own solutions. In this way, therapists were able to help clients understand for themselves what they needed and how to move forward in life. In the cultural context of the time, in which it was assumed that the therapist had the expertise on the client's mental world, it represented a challenge to the establishment of the day to consider that people might be their own best experts.

Rogers used the terms counselling and psychotherapy interchangeably, only introducing the term counselling early in his career because of objections raised by the profession of psychiatry to his use of the term psychotherapy. At the time, psychotherapy was seen as the province of psychiatry and was heavily influenced by the ideas of psychoanalysis. Rogers, as a psychologist, was therefore not seen to be offering psychotherapy in the approach that he was developing. For this reason he called it non-directive counselling. Because of this terminological heritage, some still view counselling and psychotherapy as different. However, consistent with Rogers' approach I use the terms counselling and psychotherapy interchangeably in this book with the term therapy.

Almost a decade after his 1942 book on counselling and psychotherapy, Rogers published *Client-Centered Therapy*, in which he presented his more refined ideas (Rogers, 1951). Most notably, Rogers had replaced the term *non-directive* with the term *client-centred*. Essentially, the terms non-directive and client-centred refer to opposite sides of the same coin. Whereas non-directive refers to what it is the therapist aspires *not to do*, that is to challenge the client's agency over their own feelings and perceptions, the term client-centred refers to what the therapist aspires *to do*, which is to support the agency of the client and go with their direction in terms of understanding what hurts and what is needed.

Throughout his life Rogers was a prolific researcher and writer, publishing numerous academic papers and books, many of which are still widely read today, such as his 1961 book *On Becoming a Person: A Therapist's View of Psychotherapy* published in 1961. He continued researching and writing up to his death on 4 February 1987 in San Diego, California. But the 1950s were a golden age of person-centred therapy when Carl Rogers published his most influential theoretical works (Rogers, 1957; 1959). In these 1957 and 1959 papers he outlined his ideas about human relationships and their effects on development and functioning.

The core set of ideas, presented as testable hypotheses in the positivist tradition, that he published in the 1950s remain the bedrock of the approach and what is referred to as the classic form of the therapy (Merry, 2004). From the classic viewpoint, what constitutes the core of the person-centred approach are three founding theoretical formulations: (1) the tendency towards actualization as the unitary motivation for human beings; (2) the developmental process of conditions of worth as the cause of psychopathology; and (3) the non-directive therapeutic relationship as the vehicle for releasing this tendency. These are topics that we shall meet in more detail in subsequent chapters as this book tends to be built around these three founding formulations.

Over the subsequent years, Rogers began to apply his ideas derived from client-centred therapy in other contexts, such as education, conflict resolution and encounter groups (see Kirschenbaum, 2007, for his most extensive biography). In order to recognize the broader applicability of his approach the term *person-centred* came to replace the term client-centred. When one reads the writings of Rogers on the broader applicability of person-centred theory it is clear that his was not only a vision for the practice of therapy but more generally for applied psychology, education and social policy, in which he envisaged a society in which relationships mattered. In this sense alone he was ahead of his time, but where person-centred therapy might be said to have always been a positive psychology is in the sense that it was never only concerned with alleviating distress and dysfunction but with helping people become more *fully functioning*. In this sense, Rogers was always concerned with −5 to +5.

Fully functioning was the term Rogers used to describe what it was that therapy freed people to move towards. It was not a description of the absence of negative qualities but a description of positive qualities. For example, one of the characteristics of the fully functioning person is that he or she lives in harmony with others and experiences the rewards of mutual positive regard. Another is that he or she is open to experience. I will return to the description of the fully functioning person later, but the point for now is that seen in contemporary terms, fully functioning seems synonymous with the notions of human flourishing now advocated by positive psychologists.

Over subsequent decades counselling and psychotherapy became swamped by the illness ideology in such a way that this original focus on fully functioning behaviour and experience was overshadowed by questions about its effectiveness for diagnostic categories.

Although the approach to person-centred therapy practised today remains very much influenced by Rogers and his key writings from this period around the middle of the last century, person-centred therapy is not an approach stranded in the 1950s and 1960s. There has been much theoretical and practical development in the world of person-centred therapy since. Rogers was not rigid in his own writings, often offering his ideas in a tentative way, and encouraging others to develop their own views.

Many other scholars have been involved in the discipline in subsequent years and the literature on the person-centred approach is much richer than it is possible to convey or appropriate to do so in this short book (see Cooper, O'Hara, Schmid, & Bohart, 2013 for contemporary developments). Although some of the notable scholars in the person-centred approach will be mentioned along the way, this book is focused on the interface of positive psychology and the person-centred approach and is not intended as a comprehensive overview of subsequent developments and offshoots of practice and theory. For example, other approaches include the experiential focusing approach (Gendlin, 1996), the process-experiential approach (Greenberg et al., 1993) and motivational interviewing (Miller & Rollnick, 2002). These approaches hold that the process of therapy can be helped along with the use of more directive methods than are associated with more traditional client-centred psychotherapy. Of practical interest have been the attempts to find ways of working within the person-centred framework with people whose psychological contact is at a very minimum level. Prouty (1990) developed an approach called pre-therapy that involves reflecting back to the client the counsellor's awareness of the client's external world and communication with others. Pre-therapy aims to help the client develop psychological contact in order that they can then enter more conventional therapy. Pre-therapy approaches have been used with some success in helping people suffering from problems of psychosis (Van Werde, 2005). These, and other offshoot approaches, together form a family of person-centred and experiential therapies (Sanders, 2013).

Bringing all those interested in the approach together is the World Association for Person-Centered and Experiential Psychotherapy and Counseling (WAPCEPC) which was founded in 1997. WAPCEPC is an association for the Science and Practice of Client-Centered and Experiential Psychotherapies and Counseling. The aim is to provide a world-wide forum for those professionals who have a commitment to the primary importance in therapy of the relationship between therapist and client and who also have a belief in the efficacy of the conditions and attitudes conducive to therapeutic movement first postulated by Carl Rogers, and a commitment to their active implementation within the therapeutic relationship.

One view from the family of person-centred and experiential therapies that I will elaborate on, however, is that of the process-directed approach in which the therapist may introduce various experiences for the client into the sessions, as discussed by Richard Worsley (2009).

Remarkably, over 50 years later the view that it is the client and not the therapist who knows best what direction to go in remains a powerful and revolutionary idea (see also, Duncan & Miller, 2000; Hubble & Miller, 2004) and still represents a stance which is in opposition to much of contemporary psychology, with its emphasis on expert diagnosis, formulation, treatment and interventions. As Brazier said:

> When people read about Rogers' ideas, it is not uncommon for them to think initially that there is nothing very remarkable about them. Do we not all believe in the importance of people being empathic to one another? What is so remarkable about that? What is remarkable is that Rogers actually meant it. And in carrying through what are essentially a very simple set of ideas whose rightness seems self-evident, he offers a challenge to the foundations of most of what modern life consists of. (1993, p. 8)

In summary, person-centred therapy is both a humanistic therapy in its historical context and a positive therapy in the contemporary sense of it being an example of positive psychology applied to therapy.

Positive therapy

As already noted, in the therapeutic culture of the last few decades it has been difficult for therapists to embrace the concept of fully functioning, so pervasive has the language of disorder and deficit been. The various editions of the American Psychiatric Association's Diagnostic and Statistical Manual (DSM) have for several decades now provided psychologists with the language with which to describe the ways in which people suffer. Diagnostic categories of depression, anxiety, post-traumatic stress and so on are commonly used. As a result of the pervasive influence of the psychiatric terminology the profession of therapy has become overly focused on disorder and deficit at the expense of its understandings of what leads to positive functioning (Vossler, Steffen & Joseph, 2015).

Thus, although the idea of fully functioning has been at the core of the person-centred approach for over half a century, it has only been with the advent of the contemporary positive psychology movement that psychologists have begun to look again at these ideas and to question their reliance on psychiatric terminology. As such, the ideas of Carl Rogers are now beginning to attract wider attention and to be recognized within the positive psychology literature.

However, looking in the other direction, the disciplines of counselling and psychotherapy appear increasingly distanced from the growing edge of psychological theory and research, particularly research which is not directly related to therapy, or which does not use the language of psychiatric disorders, such as that published in social, personality and developmental psychology journals, as well as the more recent positive psychology research. This has created a gap between theory and practice in counselling and psychotherapy. Many of the key training texts in humanistic therapy make only passing reference to the contemporary psychological literature (see Cooper & Joseph, in press, who make this argument).

As a result it may be a surprise to many therapists to learn that many of the ideas once associated with person-centred psychology remain at the core of some research programmes in social, personality and developmental psychology, although now often using different terminology. Specifically, the research programme into Self-Determination Theory (SDT) posits that human beings have three basic psychological needs: 'essential for facilitating optimal functioning of the natural propensities for growth and integration' (Ryan & Deci, 2000, p. 68). The first of these is a need for *relatedness* – defined as feeling connected to others; caring for, and being cared by, those others – and this sits alongside a need for *autonomy* (having a sense of agency and ownership of one's behaviour), and a need for *competence* (a sense of mastery and accomplishment).

SDT is becoming increasingly influential in the field of positive psychology as well as more widely in the fields of motivation and emotion, personality and social psychology. What is clear from close scrutiny of SDT is that its conceptualization of need satisfactions is essentially a 'positively phrased' way of expressing what person-centred therapists strive to achieve through the 'negatively phrased' concept of non-directivity. When the person-centred approach is considered in light of this other research the evidence is stronger than ever that the self-determination of the client is all-important if they are to make changes in their life, and that in fostering self-determination it is the relationship between the therapist and the client that matters (see Cooper & Joseph, in press; Patterson & Joseph, 2007a; Sheldon, 2013 for detailed reviews).

By combining Rogers' theoretical ideas, 50 years of relationship-related psychotherapy research, and the recent positive psychological research, a powerful case is made for how to alleviate distress and simultaneously facilitate human flourishing.

The above sections set the scene for the book by briefly introducing positive psychology and the person-centred approach of Carl Rogers. My argument is that the person-centred approach is a positive psychology because it is a therapy that was explicitly developed in order to facilitate fully functioning behaviour. Positive therapy emerges from the synthesis of positive psychology and person-centred therapy.

Aims of the book

1   To show the relevance of positive psychology to therapy such that therapy no longer restricts itself to the alleviation of suffering, especially as defined by psychiatric categories, but sees its purpose as the facilitation of well-being, human flourishing and optimal functioning.
2   To show that person-centred therapy is an original positive psychology because of its focus on promoting fully functioning behaviour.
3   To show how person-centred theory and therapy is underpinned by the research and philosophy of self-determination theory (SDT) and other mainstream social and developmental psychology research.
4   To show how person-centred theory provides an integrative view of positive and negative experiences, in such a way as to reconceptualize psychopathology as the thwarting of the human tendency towards flourishing.
5   To argue for the use of theory-consistent measures in research and practice (e.g., to assess authenticity) instead of and alongside the traditional measures derived from the psychiatric model.

Plan for the book

In Chapter 2 I will introduce positive psychology in more depth and how it is concerned with well-being, human flourishing and optimal functioning in the broadest sense to include all aspects of hedonic and eudaimonic well-being. Generally speaking, hedonic well-being refers to our striving for pleasure whereas eudaimonic well-being refers to our need for meaning. Even though these are related aspects of experience, the conceptual distinction is useful in focusing our minds on what the aims of therapy actually are.

In Chapter 3 I will discuss how the positive psychology movement has provided the impetus to re-examine the fundamental assumptions that underlie the professional practice of psychology. By fundamental assumptions I am referring to deep-seated beliefs that one may not always be fully aware of. Basically, my argument will be that our assumptions about human nature can be broadly grouped into one of two camps. Either, we hold that people are intrinsically motivated by constructive impulses, or we hold that people are intrinsically motivated by destructive impulses. The point is that we cannot escape how our fundamental assumptions influence us as therapists. How a therapist listens to what the person in front of them is saying is inevitably influenced by their deep-seated assumptions. I will discuss the implication of one's fundamental assumptions for therapy practice. It is my intention that readers reflect on their own assumptions and how they relate these to their own ways of working therapeutically. It is the assumption that people are intrinsically motivated in positive and socially constructive ways (the *actualizing tendency*) that forms the foundation of person-centred theory and therapy.

In Chapter 4 I continue to explore the person-centred theory of Carl Rogers, specifically his development and personality theory which posits how it is the congruence between the actualizing tendency and socialisation processes that give rise to well-being. I consider how person-centred theory appears to be consistent with what the positive psychology research is now telling us.

In Chapter 5 I describe person-centred therapy. Seen through the lens of modern positive psychology, person-centred therapy as originated by Carl Rogers offers a revolutionary and radical way of working with people. The research evidence shows that the self-determination of the client is important, and that it is the relationship between the therapist and the client that is important.

In Chapter 6 I discuss process-directed positive therapy and consider the recent positive psychological research on person-activity fit. For example, exercises in gratitude in which people are asked to reflect on the things that they are appreciative of have been found to be beneficial. I will discuss how such exercises can be used by therapists working in a person-centred way. In short, my argument is that it is not what the therapist does but how they do it that is important.

In Chapter 7 I discuss the implications of the positive psychological approach to therapy for understanding psychopathology. I argue that a genuinely positive psychological approach should speak to both the negative side of human experience as well as the positive side. I describe how the person-centred approach rejects the medical model, seeing it as irrelevant, unnecessary and not useful. The result is that we begin to understand well-being as a function of the extent of congruence between a person's intrinsic tendency toward actualization and their self-actualization, with higher levels of congruence leading to increasing well-being, and incongruence leading to psychopathology. Thus, the model recognizes that congruence is the foundation stone of both psychopathology and fulfilment.

In Chapter 8 I discuss my own work in the field of post-traumatic stress and post-traumatic growth to illustrate the positive therapy approach. I describe the organismic valuing theory of growth through adversity, which explains how positive adaptation to threatening events leads to the well-recognized processes of intrusion and avoidance that are found within post-traumatic stress. I then show that the 'completion principle' that is commonly described within theories of post-traumatic stress can be understood as part of the broader actualizing tendency, and that following this actualizing tendency leads to increases in psychological well-being and movement towards growth and being more fully functioning.

In Chapter 9 I will discuss the idea of theory-consistent measurement. As we turn to positive psychology and person-centred therapy our aim is to help people become more fully functioning, authentic, open to experience and so on. As such it is appropriate that we begin to evaluate the success of therapy in relation to these aims, rather than the absence of psychiatric disorders. For some, this is a controversial position as person-centred therapists have long questioned the use of tests to assess and diagnose clients. My argument is that the same logic does not apply to positive psychological tests which are consistent with person-centred theory and may in fact enhance the therapeutic process.

Finally, in Chapter 10 I will consider how positive therapy focuses our attention on the social and political context of our work as therapists. Put simply, we have a choice as professional psychologists to be facilitators of personal growth or to be promoters of social adjustment. Sometimes, personal growth and social adjustment are in alignment and there is no conflict, but often there is conflict. As therapists we have a choice to make: are we to foster personal growth or are we to foster social adjustment? Many of the problems of living encountered in modern society come about as a result of social forces and the demands of living in materialistic cultures. As a result, therapists have to strike a balance between social adjustment and personal transformation.

Conclusion

As the positive psychology movement takes root more widely and continues to develop, it is my hope that the aims and aspirations of the positive psychology movement will permeate the research and practice of all psychologists and therapists, thereby broadening their focus to incorporate the full range of human experience and functioning, from distress and disorder to well-being and fulfilment.

Further reading:

Mearns, D., Thorne, B., & McLeod, J. (2013). *Person-centred counselling in action* (4th ed.). London: Sage.
This is a highly regarded introduction text to the person-centred approach by some of the most influential contemporary scholars in person-centred therapy.

Peterson, C. (2007). *A primer in positive psychology*. New York: Oxford University Press.
This is one of the best introductory books on positive psychology. It is lively, accessible and fun to read, written by one the founders of positive psychology.

Rogers, C. R. (1980). *A way of being*. Boston: Houghton Mifflin.
How could there not be a book by Rogers himself in this list, but which one to choose? This is one of his later ones and one of my favourites.

Chapter 2

Positive psychology

In this chapter my aim is to introduce positive psychology. As already mentioned in the previous chapter, the beginning of positive psychology was Martin E. P. Seligman's 1998 Presidential Address to the American Psychological Association (APA) (Seligman, 1999). Seligman has told how the idea of positive psychology came to him following a moment of epiphany when gardening with his daughter Nikki who was then aged five when she instructed him not to be such a grouch. 'In that moment, I acquired the mission of helping to build the scientific infrastructure of a field that would investigate what makes life worth living: positive emotion, positive character, and positive institutions' (Seligman, 2004, p. xi).

Seligman realized that psychology had largely neglected the latter two of its three pre-World War II missions: curing mental illness, helping all people to lead more productive and fulfilling lives, and identifying and nurturing high talent (see Seligman 2002). The neglect might be seen to have begun with the advent of the United States Veterans Administration in 1946 and the United States National Institute of Mental Health (NIMH) in 1947 which largely rendered psychology a healing discipline based upon a disease model and illness ideology (Seligman & Csikszentmihalyi, 2000; see also Maddux, Snyder, & Lopez, 2004 who referring to the NIMH, joked that 'perhaps it should have been named the National Institute for mental illness', p. 323).

What Seligman realized was that when it comes to understanding problems in living, a considerable amount of time and money had been spent over the years documenting the various ways in which people suffer psychologically, as was evidenced by the various editions of the Diagnostic and Statistical Manual of Mental Disorders (DSM) produced by the American Psychiatric Association. But nowhere near the same effort had gone into understanding what makes life worth living, enjoyable and meaningful. It was with this realization that Seligman resolved to use his APA Presidency to initiate a shift in psychology's focus toward a more positive psychology.

Aims and approach of positive psychology

The presidential initiative by Seligman was catalyzed through a series of meetings with both junior and senior scholars who would become the leading voices of the new positive psychology movement, and who began to map out what they saw as a positive psychology research agenda. This was followed by the hugely influential January 2000 special issue of the *American Psychologist* on positive psychology, which was the landmark for the beginning of this new field of scholarship and practice (Seligman & Csikszentimihalyi, 2000). As Seligman and Csikszentimihalyi (2000), editors of the special issue, said:

> The aim of positive psychology is to begin to catalyze a change in the focus of psychology from preoccupation only with repairing the worst things in life to also building positive qualities. (p. 5)

This 'special issue on happiness, excellence, and optimal human functioning' included articles on individual development, subjective well-being, optimism, self-determination theory, adaptive mental mechanisms, emotions and health, wisdom, excellence, creativity, giftedness and positive youth development, thereby providing a broad vista of topics that were deemed to be covered under the positive psychology umbrella.

The new positive psychology contrasted very much with the more traditional emphasis by psychologists on illness and psychopathology. Although there have always been scholars interested in positive human functioning (e.g., Andrews & Withey, 1976), most professional psychologists had traditionally earned their living by helping people to cope better with their problems rather than helping people to live their life to the full. As such, psychologists were well versed in the treatment of various so-called disorders and how to help people reduce their levels of distress and dysfunction, but when it came to helping people live to the full, they were at a loss to know how to help. The aim of positive psychology was to revolutionize how professional psychologists thought about what they were doing, so that their work was not only about the alleviation of distress and dysfunction, but also about the promotion of well-being and optimal functioning.

The field of positive psychology quickly took off. From the outset there was the publication of several major handbooks (e.g., Linley & Joseph, 2004a; Peterson & Seligman, 2004; Snyder & Lopez, 2002), introductory texts (e.g., Bolt, 2004; Carr, 2003; Compton, 2004), a number of edited volumes dealing with a variety of positive psychology topics (e.g., Aspinwall & Staudinger, 2003; Cameron, Dutton, & Quinn, 2003; Keyes & Haidt, 2002; Lopez & Snyder, 2003), and many journal special issues or special sections – all of which helped to quickly establish the new field. A new dedicated journal was also soon introduced, *The Journal of Positive Psychology* (see Linley, Joseph, Harrington, & Wood, 2006, for a review of the emergence of positive psychology).

The role of the practitioner, from a positive psychological perspective, is not only to alleviate distress but also how to facilitate well-being, promote health and build strengths. The ideas of positive psychology have been applied widely in many domains of life. For example, the questions of happiness as a public policy aim (Veenhoven, 2004); the benefit of national indicators of subjective well-being (Diener & Seligman, 2004; Pavot & Diener, 2004); the need to understand the optimal experiences of disabled people, rather than simply seeing them as 'disabled' (Delle Fave & Massimini, 2004); working with offenders in ways that recognize their needs and aspirations, thereby significantly reducing recidivism (Ward & Mann, 2004); the need to balance individuality and community in order to achieve good lives for all (Myers, 2004); and the opportunity of being able to prevent disorder and promote well-being through population-based approaches (Huppert, 2004). These initiatives are united by their positive psychological approach to the issues that are of concern. For many in mainstream psychology at the time these were genuinely new ways of thinking that challenged decades of research and practice.

Methods of positive psychology

At the outset the leaders of the positive psychology movement emphasized that while the topics might be new, the scientific methods of psychology were still just as applicable. As Sheldon and King (2001) said:

> What is positive psychology? It is nothing more than the scientific study of ordinary human strengths and virtues. Positive psychology revisits 'the average person,' with an interest in finding out what works, what is right, and what is improving. (p. 216)

Scientific methods such as experimentation allow important questions about positive psychology to be answered with empirical sophistication. The body of knowledge in positive psychology has grown considerably through the use of such methods. Many of the initial hypotheses that were set up in the early years of positive psychology are now tested, giving us the evidence needed to take positive psychology beyond conjecture. For example, confirming hypotheses about the personal benefits of living one's life in such a way as to regularly use one's strengths of character, Niemiec (2013) found that presence of character strengths is strongly associated with higher levels of well-being and lower levels of psychological distress. Likewise, various positive interventions have also now been shown to boost happiness. For example, one of the most widely cited interventions is the counting your blessings exercise where people are asked to write down, just before going to sleep, three things that went well that day, now known to be effective in increasing well-being (Seligman, Steen, Park, & Peterson, 2005; Sin & Lyubomirsky, 2009).

The emphasis on scientific methods has served positive psychology well in establishing itself as a credible discipline in the eyes of mainstream academics in the psychological sciences and research funding bodies. However, as positive psychology has matured it has become increasingly recognized that human experience is at the core of positive psychology and as such there are questions that we might want to ask that experimental methods struggle to answer. As Rathunde (2001) noted, researchers can also learn much from the 'experiential turns' of such early psychological pioneers as James, Dewey and Maslow, who focused on immediate subjective experience in trying to understand optimal human fulfilment. While it is still true that positive psychology favours experimental methods, the questions that positive psychologists ask may sometimes be beyond their remit.

We should not thereby exclude the questions as not worth asking, but should rather seek to answer them in the most appropriate way that we can. The growing array of qualitative methodologies (e.g., interpretative phenomenological analysis; grounded theory; discourse analysis) may also lead to insights into other aspects of human experience. As such there is a growing trend within positive psychology to develop research using these methods as well. As such, positive psychology is now open to both quantitative and qualitative methods in its explorations of well-being and human functioning.

Range of positive psychology

As already noted, since its inception the range of topics of interest to positive psychologists has been broad, and these have continued to expand to include new areas of application, such as curiosity, gratitude, forgiveness, post-traumatic growth, meaning and purpose in life, to name but a few research topics which have gained attention. New areas of application have also opened up as positive psychologists influence other areas such as health, education and social policy (Joseph, 2015). In essence, the ideas of positive psychology seem to be applicable to every domain of life that involves human behaviour.

The appeal of positive psychology continues to grow. Since the first edition of this book there has been the publication of several new textbooks (e.g., Hefferon & Boniwell, 2011; Peterson, 2006; Snyder & Lopez, 2007) and specialist books (e.g., Csikszentmihalyi & Csikszentmihalyi, 2006; David, Boniwell, & Conley Ayers, 2013; Joseph & Linley, 2008a). There are now biannual conferences organized by the *International Positive Psychology Association* (IPPA) and the *European Network for Positive Psychology* (ENPP), together with a host of conference themes and sections dedicated to positive psychology in other areas of psychology. For example, and of particular relevance to this book, the Society of Counseling Psychology, states that their 'philosophy emphasizes developmental, strength-based, multicultural, and social justice principles, as well as positive psychology and international perspectives' (American Psychological Association, 2013). As such, positive psychology is now mentioned as part of what defines counselling psychology as a profession.

While some might have seen positive psychology as a passing fad, it is now well established and its influence on practice will continue to grow. Nonetheless there have been critics along the way.

Criticism of positive psychology

Early on in the development of positive psychology, a criticism was that positive psychology emphasized the 'positive' at the expense of the 'negative' (Held, 2002;

Lazarus, 2003). While this may have been true initially, I do not believe it remains a justifiable concern. There is now a substantial move within positive psychology that emphasizes the integration of the positive and negative (e.g., Pauwels, 2015). Certainly, there is the recognition that we need more understanding of the positive but this should not be at the expense of the negative, and indeed, an understanding of positive states may even help us to work more effectively with negative states. Research shows that the facilitation of well-being is not only a worthwhile goal in its own right but may actually serve a preventative function against future psychopathology (e.g., Fredrickson, 1998; 2001; Fredrickson & Levenson, 1998; Wood & Joseph, 2010).

The focus of research should be on understanding the entire breadth of human experience, from loss, suffering, illness and distress through connection, fulfilment, health and well-being. This is especially relevant for therapeutic contexts, since the role of the therapist remains first and foremost to alleviate distress and dysfunction.

Levels of analysis

Positive psychology is also concerned with all levels of human functioning, from the person through to larger institutions. As Gable and Haidt (2005) said:

> Positive psychology is the study of the conditions and processes that contribute to the flourishing or optimal functioning of people, groups, and institutions. (p. 104)

Likewise, Seligman and Csikszentmihalyi (2000) said:

> The field of positive psychology at the subjective level is about valued subjective experiences: well-being, contentment, and satisfaction (in the past); hope and optimism (for the future); and flow and happiness (in the present). At the individual level, it is about positive individual traits: the capacity for love and vocation, courage, interpersonal skill, aesthetic sensibility, perseverance, forgiveness, originality, future mindedness, spirituality, high talent, and wisdom. At the group level, it is about the civic virtues and the institutions that move individuals toward better citizenship: responsibility, nurturance, altruism, civility, moderation, tolerance, and work ethic. (p. 5)

Two types of well-being

In the section above the term well-being was mentioned several times. One of the most important developments since the beginnings of positive psychology has been the philosophical consideration of the question of what is good and desirable within positive psychology and the meaning of well-being.

Throughout the literature, a number of authors have drawn a distinction both empirically and theoretically between two general philosophical perspectives, the eudaimonic and the hedonic (see Ryan & Deci, 2001; Huta & Waterman, 2014; Keyes, Shmotkin, & Ryff, 2002).

A hedonic orientation involves seeking happiness, positive affect, life satisfaction, and reduced negative affect. In this way hedonia refers to an absence of distress or an affective balance such that positive experiences outweigh negative experiences.

Various definitions of eudaimonia exist. A recent view is provided by Huta and Waterman (2014) who argue that four core definitional elements appeared across most definitions. First, *authenticity*, which refers to clarifying one's true self and deep values, staying connected with them, and acting in accord with them. Second, *meaning*, which refers to understanding a bigger picture that provides a sense of identity, purpose and an understanding of how one is connected to others, society, the ecosystem. Third, *excellence*, which refers to striving for higher quality and higher standards in one's behaviour, performance, accomplishments and ethics. Fourth, *growth*, which refers to actualizing one's potential, and pursuing personal goals, learning, and seeking new challenges so that one matures as a human being (see Huta, 2015, for a detailed review).

In essence, hedonia is about pleasure in life, whereas eudaimonia is about meaning. The two types of well-being are typically moderately correlated (Compton, Smith, Cornish, & Qualls, 1996; Keyes et al., 2002; Waterman, 1993). Indeed, some of the most fulfilling activities in life are the ones where hedonia and eudaimonia are so seamlessly blended that they become one. Nonetheless, this should not be taken to mean that they are largely synonymous (Huta & Ryan, 2010). The different implications of these two different types of well-being for positive psychology are important.

There are two ways of thinking about hedonia and eudaimonia. First, we can see these as the experiences we have. Second, we can see these as orientations, in the sense that each of us prioritizes activities in our life that more incline us in one direction or the other (Huta & Waterman, 2014; Huta, 2015). In this second sense we can consider our motives for our own behaviour, whether for example we are engaging in activities to enhance pleasure or to find meaning. Similarly, we can also think about our goals as therapists – whether for our clients we wish to enhance their pleasure or meaning.

Traditionally psychologists have thought of their task as alleviating psychological suffering. With positive psychology we begin to think about facilitating well-being. But given this distinction we then have to ask ourselves what type of well-being do we mean? Do we wish to promote hedonic or eudaimonic well-being?

Subjective and psychological well-being

In contemporary literature these two forms of well-being, the hedonic and the eudaimonic, are referred to as subjective well-being (SWB) and psychological well-being

(PWB), respectively. Important distinctions arise between people who have much pleasure in life but are unfulfilled (i.e., high SWB, low PWB) and between people who may not be perceived as 'happy' but who find their lives deeply meaningful (i.e., low SWB, high PWB). Then there are those who have both pleasure and meaning in their lives (high SWB, high PWB) and those who have neither (low SWB and low PWB).

The implications of the distinction for practice are considerable. Questions have been raised over SWB as the sole pursuit. If SWB were the sole goal of positive psychology, should we sanction ever-greater experience of momentary positive affect and avoidance of negative affect? We know from personal experience that when we want to boost our mood we are often drawn towards ways to increase our momentary hedonic states. Yet, the evidence clearly indicates the contrary: more money, more materialism and more possessions – the things that many of us feel inclined towards when we want to boost our happiness – actually all fail to make us any happier in the longer term (Csikszentmihalyi, 1999; Kasser, 2015).

In fact, such materialistic pursuits may have even the reverse effect, leading to psychological ill-being (Kasser, 2015; Kasser & Ryan, 1993; 1996) and greater ecological costs that are a detriment to our long-term environmental well-being and survival (Sheldon & McGregor, 2000). The pursuit of ever more SWB is likely to be personally, socially and environmentally unsustainable (Sheldon & McGregor, 2000).

In contrast, recent evidence suggests that greater PWB is related to better SWB. Wood and Joseph (2010) investigated the effect of low PWB on the onset of clinical depression in a sample of over 5,500 people over a 10-year period in a sample of people aged 55–56. People low in PWB were over seven times more likely to meet clinical cut-offs for depression 10 years later. With very conservative control variables (including initial depression, personality, demographic, economic and physical health variables) people with low PWB were still more than twice as likely to be depressed 10 years later.

Not surprisingly then, the last decade has seen a shift in positive psychology from an almost exclusive focus on SWB to a more nuanced and balanced view of well-being that accommodates both SWB and PWB perspectives.

Such personal transformation in terms of greater PWB is not the traditional concern of psychological therapists whose concern has been more likely to be with increasing SWB (i.e. lower depression, anxiety, negative affect, greater happiness, relaxation, positive affectivity, etc.). Of course, in the sense that clients come to therapy because they are feeling unhappy then all therapies are concerned with SWB, but the point that I am making is that whereas many traditional therapies aim to directly increase SWB by introducing exercises to help the person think differently so as to feel better, positive psychology challenges us to also consider PWB as an aim of therapy.

Positive psychotherapy

As positive psychology has gathered attention, there has been interest in its application to psychotherapy. In the section below I will briefly describe some of the main therapeutic approaches that have come to be considered under the umbrella of positive psychotherapies. It is not my intention to provide a comprehensive review but to give the flavour of some of the developments in order that readers can contrast these approaches with the person-centred approach to positive therapy.

Positive psychotherapy (PPT)

PPT is based on Seligman's theory of authentic happiness (Seligman, 2003b; Seligman, Rashid & Parks, 2008) and is a prescriptive therapy that involves the client engaging in various exercises over three phases. First, the client explores their signature strengths which are then operationalized into personally meaningful goals. The middle phase focuses on cultivating positive emotions and adaptively dealing with negative memories. Finally, the client is encouraged to focus on fostering positive relationships and meaning and purpose. For example, in session 1 the client is asked to tell a story about them at their best, and to complete a questionnaire to assess their strengths, and to think of ways in which to use their strengths more often. In session 2 clients discuss their strengths and at home complete an online questionnaire and have friends and family identify their strengths. Over the sessions clients work through a series of such exercises that target different strengths, until the final session when there is discussion about how to sustain strengths beyond therapy (Rashid, 2015a).

The theoretical rationale underpinning this is that using one's strengths conveys a sense of ownership and authenticity in their use, because people feel an intrinsic yearning to use them and a feeling of inevitability in doing so. Hence, using one's signature strengths is considered to be concordant with one's intrinsic interests and values (Peterson & Seligman, 2004). Further, Peterson and Seligman suggest that the use of strengths will bring about tangible outcomes, such as subjective well-being, competence, efficacy, mastery, mental health and rich social networks. Hence, using one's signature strengths is considered to serve well-being and basic psychological needs, such as competence, autonomy, relatedness and self-esteem. In this way, using one's strengths is considered to act as a buffer against mental illness (Seligman & Peterson, 2003). Several pilot studies have applied PPT to treat symptoms of depression, anxiety, psychosis, borderline personality disorder, and to support smoking cessation (see Rashid, 2015a for a summary).

Well-being therapy

Well-being therapy was developed by Fava and colleagues (e.g. Fava, 1997; 1999; Ruini & Fava, 2004), based on Ryff's (e.g., 1989; Ryff & Singer, 1996) research on the six identified domains of psychological well-being, namely environmental mastery, personal growth, purpose in life, autonomy, self-acceptance and positive relations with others. Well-being therapy is described as a short-term psychotherapeutic strategy that extends over eight sessions, with each session ranging from 30 to 50 minutes. It emphasizes self-observation, including the use of a structured diary, and the interaction between the client and the therapist (Ruini & Fava, 2004, p. 374).

Fava (2000) recognized that cognitive-behavioural therapies had impressive track records in symptom reduction, but were lacking in their complete resolution of psychopathology. Ruini and Fava (2004) identified four reasons that provided the context for the development of well-being therapy. First, there has been increasing awareness of relapse in affective disorders, especially unipolar major depression. While therapeutic intervention may remove the symptoms for a time, the effects are not particularly long-lasting. Second, concerns of residual symptomatology, such as anxiety, irritability and interpersonal problems, have often been found to characterize patients who were in remission according to DSM criteria, but who were nonetheless still far from well-functioning. Third, increasing interest in quality of life assessment in health care has placed these questions more squarely on the clinical agenda. Fourth, the growth of positive psychology has brought to bear positive psychological perspectives on clinical populations, further driving the need for the promotion of well-being, rather than just the alleviation of symptomatology.

Recognizing this, Fava (e.g. 1999) sought to build on existing cognitive-behavioural frameworks but also to incorporate a focus on the facilitation of well-being, in the belief that improvements in well-being would serve to buffer against subsequent psychopathology, thereby countering relapse, reducing residual symptomatology, and improving global functioning and psychological well-being. Using Ryff's framework of psychological well-being (e.g., Ryff & Singer, 1996), which includes the six dimensions of environmental mastery, personal growth, purpose in life, autonomy, self-acceptance and positive relations with others, the client is helped to identify areas of their psychological well-being that may be improved. The therapist then proceeds to work with the client on these areas, as well as on the presenting symptoms of disorder.

During the initial session, the client is asked to identify episodes of well-being and locate them in their situational context, no matter how short lived they were. During the intermediate sessions, the client is encouraged to identify the thoughts and beliefs that lead to the premature interruption of well-being, but with the trigger for self-observation being based on well-being, rather than distress. The therapist uses this information to identify specific impairments in well-being, and then works with the client to repair these. The therapist may also choose to use self-rating inventories, such as Ryff's (1989) Psychological Well-Being Scales, to assist with the identification of problematic well-being areas. This information then paves the way for more specific well-being enhancement strategies.

To date, well-being therapy has been used very effectively with people suffering from a range of clinical disorders, including affective disorders (Fava, Rafanelli, Cazzaro, et al., 1998), recurrent depression (Fava, Rafanelli, Grandi, et al., 1998), loss of clinical effect (Fava, Ruini, Rafanelli, & Grandi, 2002), and generalized anxiety disorder (Fava et al., 2005; for a fuller discussion, see Ruine & Fava, 2015).

Mindfulness-based cognitive therapy

Mindfulness has long been recognized as a means for improving self-awareness, and thereby allowing one to make more informed and deliberate choices. Empirical work from the positive psychology tradition has shown how mindfulness is associated with a host of well-being indicators (Brown & Ryan, 2003). It has also been shown that mindfulness-based approaches provide possible means of fostering self-determination and self-awareness, and in this way allow the satisfaction of basic psychological needs for autonomy, competence and relatedness (see Brown & Ryan, 2004; Brown & Ryan, 2003), which are believed to underpin much of human well-being (Ryan & Deci, 2000).

Within therapeutic settings, mindfulness training has been allied with cognitive-behavioural therapy in order to try and prevent the problems of relapse following treatment for depression that were described above. According to Teasdale et al. (2000), vulnerability to relapse and recurrence of depression arises from the fact that the person makes repeated associations between their depressed mood and patterns of negative, self-devaluing, hopeless thinking during episodes of major depression. This leads to changes at both the cognitive and neuronal levels, such that people who have experienced major depression, but who have recovered, differ from people who have never experienced major depression in their patterns of thinking that are triggered by low mood or dysphoria.

The focus of mindfulness-based cognitive therapy is then to teach individuals to become aware of how thoughts and feelings relate to them in a wider, decentred perspective. In this way, people are encouraged to view their thoughts as 'mental events' that are detached from, rather than an integral part of, the person and their psychological make-up. This detachment then provides individuals with the skills and abilities they need in order to prevent the escalation of depressive thoughts and feelings into full-blown major depression. There is growing evidence to support the effectiveness of this approach (see e.g., Teasdale et al., 2000; 2002; Ma & Teasdale, 2004) and for its use with a variety of clinical as well as non-clinical conditions (Grossman et al., 2004). Mindfulness has also been developed separately as a therapeutic approach (Segal, Williams & Teasdale, 2002; Baer, 2003) and similarly involves a non-judgemental approach to engaging with one's inner experiencing. Bishop et al. (2004), in their operational definition, propose that mindfulness encompasses two elements: *self-regulation of attention* (moment-to moment awareness) and an attitude of *curiosity, openness and acceptance towards one's experiences* including thoughts, perceptions, emotions and sensations, while Kabat-Zinn defines the approach as, *paying attention in a particular way: on purpose, in the present moment, and non-judgmentally* (Kabat-Zinn, 1994, p. 4; see also Kabat-Zinn, 2013).

Solution-focused therapy

Solution-focused therapy (O'Connell, 2005) is based on helping clients to achieve their preferred outcomes through the evocation and co-construction of solutions to their problems. Solution-focused therapy arose from the work of Steve de Shazer and his team at the Brief Family Therapy Center in Milwaukee, United States, on brief therapy. While there is some debate as to what constitutes 'brief therapy', there is an emerging consensus that brief therapy involves less than 20 sessions (O'Connell, 2005).

There is considerable agreement about what are the main characteristics of brief therapy, and perusing them shows their commonality with much of what we are describing within the framework of positive therapy. For example, Barret-Kruse (1994) summarized some of the main features of solution-focused brief therapy as the view that oneself and others are essentially able; the therapist's acceptance of the client's definition of the problem; the formation of the therapeutic alliance; and the client being credited for therapeutic success, while the therapist also learns from the client. She does also suggest that this process requires a degree of directivity from the therapist, thus locating this approach among the more process-oriented positive therapies.

Clinical approaches to post-traumatic growth

In their discussion of how clinicians may work with people following trauma in such a way that promotes and facilitates the person's capacity for growth and positive change, Tedeschi and Calhoun (2004; Calhoun & Tedeschi, 1999) are explicit in noting that therapy that seeks to facilitate post-traumatic growth is always client-led, moving at the client's pace and in the client's direction. The therapist acts as a co-traveller who, when appropriate, may note certain developments or offer alternative interpretations.

Tedeschi and Calhoun (2004) suggest six general considerations for the therapist to bear in mind when working to facilitate post-traumatic growth. These are very much consistent with my understanding of positive therapy, and so I will elaborate them a little here. First, Tedeschi and Calhoun remind the therapist that they should be working from the framework of the trauma survivor, striving to understand the client's way of thinking rather than imposing their own views, values and beliefs. Second, they commend the value of effective listening, and suggest that therapists should listen without necessarily trying to resolve the client's issues for them. Third, they suggest the therapist listens for and labels the themes of post-traumatic growth, but always with this process being led by the client, rather than directed by the therapist. Fourth, the therapist should focus on the struggle rather than the trauma; the growth that may come is a result of this struggle and adaptation, rather than a result of the trauma per se. Fifth, trauma survivors may be able to learn much from others who have experienced similar events, and as such, group approaches to the facilitation of post-traumatic growth merit consideration (see the consideration of these in Chapter 8). Finally, helping the client to engage with a developing narrative about their struggle, and to monitor their changing beliefs following the trauma can act as triggers for the recognition and celebration of growth, but as ever, only if done at the client's pace and from the client's perspective (see Tedeschi, Calhoun, & Groleau, 2015, for further elaboration).

Motivational interviewing

Motivational interviewing (MI) (Rollnick & Miller, 1995) is based on the finding that the person-centred qualities of the therapist were important ingredients of therapy, but adds a more process-directive element by skilfully helping the client to explore the pros and cons of change in order to motivate the client towards making the necessary changes. Motivational interviewing has been described as a brief and directive technique-driven form of person-centred therapy. Csillik (2013) discusses the theoretical convergence between MI and person-centred therapy, concluding that there is much overlap, and that Rogers' theory offers a potential theoretical foundation for MI in helping to understand the processes involved in MI effectiveness.

All of these therapies, in contrast to the person-centred approach, as we have already discussed, are directive to a greater or lesser extent in terms of the therapist's intent towards the client. Each of them has an agenda for the client to change in a specified direction. We will return to this theme in the next chapter, but for the moment it is useful to go back a few decades and consider positive psychology in the historical context of humanistic psychology.

Building bridges to humanistic psychology

The success of positive psychology is not in doubt, but it is also quite clear from examination of the scholarly literature that positive psychology did not 'begin' in 1998, or 1999, or 2000. Research into positive psychology topics had gone on for decades before, and might even be traced back to the origins of psychology itself, for example, in William James' writings on 'healthy mindedness' (James, 1902), through to the more contemporary work in the 1980s on happiness and life satisfaction by Michael Argyle in the United Kingdom and Ed Diener in the USA. But Seligman, Csikszentmihalyi and their colleagues achieved something quite remarkable by how they shifted the agenda of mainstream psychology to take such work more seriously, and to bring together with a common purpose an otherwise disparate collection of scholars.

To humanistic psychologists, however, these new ideas of positive psychology were not so new (e.g., see Robbins, 2015; Schneider, 2011). The big idea to shift the agenda to take more seriously what makes life worth living echoed the arguments of the humanistic psychologists several decades before. Humanistic psychology developed around the middle of the twentieth century in part to address the fact that the previous ways of thinking in psychoanalysis and behaviourism had not been concerned with the full range of functioning. As Sutich and Vich (1969), editors of the influential *Readings in Humanistic Psychology*, wrote:

> Two main branches of psychology – behaviourism and psychoanalysis – appear to have made great contributions to human knowledge, but neither singly nor together have they covered the almost limitless scope of human behaviour, relationships, and possibilities. Perhaps their greatest limitation has been the inadequacy of their approach to *positive* human potentialities and the maximal realization of those potentialities. (p. 1)

Likewise, John Shlien, a Harvard psychologist and one of the early pioneers of person-centred psychology, originally writing in 1956, said:

> In the past, mental health has been a 'residual' concept – the absence of disease. We need to do more than describe improvement in terms of say 'anxiety reduction'. We need to say what the person can *do* as health is achieved. As the emphasis on pathology lessons, there have been a few recent efforts toward positive conceptulizations of mental health. Notable among these are Carl Rogers' 'Fully Functioning Person', A. Maslow's 'Self-Realizing Persons'. (Schlien, 2003a, p. 17)

As such, while Seligman is credited with introducing the positive psychology movement it is clear from the above comments by Schlien in 1956 and by Sutich and Vich in 1969 that this theme of positive functioning was already well-trodden territory by humanistic psychologists. Indeed, even the term positive psychology had been used. The final chapter of Maslow's 1954 book, *Motivation and Personality*, was titled 'Toward a Positive Psychology', where he called for greater attention to both the positive and negative aspects of human experience: As Maslow (1954) wrote:

> The science of psychology has been far more successful on the negative than on the positive side. It has revealed to us much about man's shortcomings, his illness, his sins, but little about his potentialities, his virtues, his achievable aspirations, or his full psychological height. It is as if psychology has voluntarily restricted itself to only half its rightful jurisdiction, and that, the darker, meaner half. (p. 354)

Maslow seems to be the first to use the term positive psychology. Maslow wanted to create a psychology that was based not only on those who were dysfunctional but also upon those who were fully living the extent of their human potential. As such, there is a clear lineage between the early humanistic psychologists and the later positive psychologists.

Initially, positive psychology may not have paid sufficient tribute to its lineage from humanistic psychology (e.g., Taylor, 2001). For some in the positive psychology movement this may have been a deliberate strategy of distancing themselves from what was seen as a previous movement that had lost its way, and ultimately failed by engaging with spiritual and supernatural practices and abandoning the rigour of science.

What perhaps some positive psychologists failed to understand is that humanistic psychology is a very broad church. Person-centred psychology is part of humanistic psychology but it is not synonymous with humanistic psychology. Perhaps there is some truth in the positive psychologists' negative portrayal when one looks at some aspects of humanistic psychology. But the early pioneers of humanistic psychology such as Rogers were without doubt serious scholars. As we have seen, Rogers was dedicated to research, known for his empirical approach and for his saying that the 'facts are friendly' – his way of making the point that we should be led by evidence in an open minded yet critical way. Rogers' theoretical work was presented in the leading scientific psychology journals, such as his statement about the relationship conditions that facilitate personal growth (Rogers, 1957) or his theory of personality (Rogers, 1959). These were certainly presented as empirically testable hypotheses.

But not all those who followed in humanistic psychology took a scientific approach, and the reputation of humanistic psychology within mainstream psychology suffered. As such, perhaps it was a politically astute move by the positive psychologists to initially distance themselves from humanistic psychology. To be taken seriously by mainstream funding bodies and scholars required distancing from the perceived embarrassments of humanistic psychology. Indeed, this is likely one of the reasons why the early proponents of positive psychology advocated the use of scientific methods so strongly. What positive psychologists were able to bring to the ideas of earlier theorists such as Maslow and Rogers were the research techniques of current mainstream psychology (see Sheldon & Kasser, 2001). Forty or more years ago, when humanistic psychology was more mainstream than it is today, and these ideas were in popular currency, the methodological and statistical sophistication was not available to fully test the theories. Now, we have sophisticated techniques that allow us to run statistical analyses in seconds that would have previously taken years, and the ability to test complicated multivariate models where we examine the summative and interactive effects of many different variables at once. At the same time, as I have said, as positive psychology has become established there is now seen to be room for the introduction of more qualitative research studies to complement the quantitative, thus bringing the disciplines of humanistic and positive psychology even closer.

There may be some aspects of humanistic psychology that remain difficult to reconcile with positive psychology but this is not the case with the person-centred approach developed by Rogers. In my own work over the past decade I have tried to show how positive psychology can learn much from this earlier theory, research and practice:

> Humanistic psychology is a broad church, and there are parts of it we would not recognize as positive psychology; but in our view, the ideas of the main humanistic psychology writers . . . deserve to be set center stage within positive psychology. Theirs was an empirical stance, explicitly research based. . . . We ought to respect this lineage, and we encourage those who are not familiar with this earlier work to visit it. (Joseph & Linley, 2004, p. 365)

Although some scholars continue to argue for the independence of humanistic and positive psychology (Waterman, 2013), such voices are now the exception. As the positive psychology movement has evolved, its leaders now acknowledge that positive psychology builds upon the earlier pioneering work of, among others, Rogers and Maslow (Seligman et al., 2005). Indeed, a quick glance through the various text books on positive psychology that have appeared over the past few years show no reluctance to now acknowledge the early humanistic psychologists. Today, one only had to open any of the leading texts on positive psychology to see the theoretical lineage to humanistic psychology openly acknowledged. As Hefferon and Boniwell (2011), authors of one of the more recent textbooks, wrote:

> We truly believe that in order to understand where we are in positive psychology we have to know where we have come from. (p. 10)

It is however important to recognize that although it is true to say that the pioneers of humanistic psychology had these same views about the importance of studying the good life decades before, it was only with the new momentum of modern positive psychology that these ideas really began to take hold in the imagination of contemporary scholars and helping professionals.

Conclusion

This chapter has provided an introduction to positive psychology and the idea that we should be equally concerned with what makes life worth living as we are with what goes wrong. It is a perspective associated with positive psychology, but also an idea that dates back to the pioneering humanistic psychologists. In the next chapter we will begin to examine the ideas of humanistic psychology, and specifically the therapeutic approach of Carl Rogers.

Further reading

Seligman, M. E. P., & Csikszentmihalyi, M. (2000). Positive psychology: An introduction. *American Psychologist, 55*, 5–14.
This is the special issue that started it all, so a good place to begin.

Seligman, M. E. P., Steen, T. A., Park, N., & Peterson, C. (2005). Positive psychology progress: Empirical validation of interventions. *American Psychologist, 60*, 410–421.
Seligman, M. E. P., Rashid, T., & Parks, A. C. (2008). Positive psychotherapy. *American Psychologist, 61*, 774–788.
Two further important papers that have paved the way for the development of positive psychology and its application to therapy.

Lopez, S. J., & Snyder, C. R. (2009). *Oxford handbook of positive psychology*. New York: Oxford University Press.
The seminal reference book containing 65 chapters from leading scholars and practitioners in positive psychology.

Joseph, S. *Positive psychology in practice: Promoting human flourishing in work, health, education, and everyday life* (2nd ed.). Hoboken, NJ: Wiley.
This handbook complements the above book by providing coverage of the applications of positive therapy.

Chapter 3

The actualizing tendency

It is not possible to live as a human being without having an idea of what it is to be human. (Heelas & Lock, 1981, p. 3)

Two therapists are listening to their client. To an outside observer both may just look as if they are doing the same thing. But the two therapists may be listening in very different ways indeed. In this chapter the paradigmatic difference between therapists, depending on their fundamental assumptions about human nature will be described. Ultimately, the practice of therapy rests on the ontology – the understanding of the nature of being. The aim of this chapter is to reflect on the fundamental assumptions of therapy and to describe the actualizing tendency which is the assumption that underpins person-centred therapy.

The ghost in the machine

In my view the most important decision a therapist can ever make is their ontological position. All therapists need a clear, coherent and consistent view of human nature. One of the most beneficial aspects of positive psychology has been its invitation to us to reflect on this question. Seligman, the champion of positive psychology, said:

There has been a profound obstacle to a science and practice of positive traits and positive states: the belief that virtue and happiness are inauthentic, epiphenomenal, parasitic upon or reducible to the negative traits and states. This 'rotten-to-the-core' view pervades Western thought, and if there is any doctrine positive psychology seeks to overthrow it is this one. Its original manifestation is the doctrine of original sin. In secular form, Freud dragged this doctrine into 20th-century psychology where it remains fashionably entrenched in academia today. For Freud, all of civilization is just an elaborate defence against basic conflicts over infantile sexuality and aggression. (2003a, p. 126)

As Seligman (2003a) said, much of modern psychology has been dominated by the doctrine of Freud, 'the ghost in the machine' of psychology and psychotherapy. Positive psychology made explicit the fact that the practice of psychology had traditionally rested on a fundamental assumption that emphasized human nature as negative in orientation and needing to be controlled (see Hubble & Miller, 2004; Maddux, 2002; Maddux, Snyder & Lopez, 2004). If Seligman is right and this view pervades Western academic thought, then we must accept that much of what goes on in the name of professional psychology is about 'cutting out the rotten bits'.

Positive psychology showed that mainstream psychology rested on a fundamental assumption that human nature is essentially destructive. Yet rarely do psychologists stop and reflect on where and why this view arose. Is it true that people are 'rotten-to-the-core'? I would argue that the evidence just does not point this way, and although it is true that people inflict much pain and suffering on each other, there are other explanations for this that do not require us to adopt the assumption that people are 'rotten-to-the-core'.

Having discarded the 'rotten-to-the-core' view of human nature, positive psychologists are now casting around for new ways of conceptualizing human nature. Fortunately, psychology has a very rich heritage of ideas, and when we look into the past of the discipline we find that the questions we are now asking are ones that many of the greatest psychologists have also tackled. Two such psychologists are Karen Horney and Carl Rogers.

Karen Horney on human nature

One of the first psychologists of the modern age to make the nature of our fundamental assumptions explicit was Karen Horney. In considering how views of human nature influenced our perspective on the promotion of living a good life (or a *morality of evolution*), Horney (1951) delineated three possible positions in trying to understand core human nature. The first position was that people are by nature sinful or driven by primitive instincts. This first perspective accords with the 'rotten-to-the-core' view that we have just discussed. The second position was that, inherent within human nature, was a mix of both something essentially destructive and something essentially constructive. From this second position, the goal of society is to ensure that the 'good' side of human nature triumphs over the 'bad' side. The third position was that inherent within people are evolutionary constructive forces which guide people towards realizing their potentialities.

Horney was careful to note that this third position did *not* suggest that people were inherently good (since this would presuppose knowledge of what constitutes good and bad). Rather, the person's values would arise from their striving towards their potential, and these values would thus be constructive and prosocial in their nature (and hence may be considered 'good'). From this third position, the goal of society is therefore to cultivate the facilitative social-environmental conditions that are conducive to people's self-realization. When people's tendency toward self-realization is allowed expression, Horney argued that:

we become free to grow ourselves, we also free ourselves to love and to feel concern for other people. We will then want to give them the opportunity for unhampered growth when they are young, and to help them in whatever way possible to find and realize themselves when they are blocked in their development. At any rate, whether for ourselves or for others, the ideal is the liberation and cultivation of the forces which lead to self-realization. (1951, pp. 15–16)

The above quote from Horney captures the essence of this book – how within people there is an urge towards self-realization. As I already said I believe the most important practical decision any therapist can make is deciding on their ontological position. Likewise, as Yalom (2001) writes:

> When I was finding my way as a young psychotherapy student, the most useful book I read was Karen Horney's *Neurosis and Human Growth*. And the single most useful concept in that book was the notion that the human being has an inbuilt propensity toward self-realization. If obstacles are removed, Horney believed, the individual will develop into a mature, fully realized adult, just as an acorn will develop into an oak tree. 'Just as an acorn develops into an oak . . . ' What a wonderful liberating and clarifying image! It forever changed my approach to psychotherapy by offering me a new vision of my work: My task was to remove obstacles blocking my patient's path. I did not have to do the entire job; I did not have to inspirit the patient with the desire to grow, with curiosity, will, zest for life, caring, loyalty, or any of the myriad of characteristics that make us fully human. No, what I had to do was to identify and remove obstacles. The rest would follow automatically, fueled by the self-actualizing forces within the patient. (p. 1)

This quote from Yalom captures the ontological position that was taken by Carl Rogers who is the person who has done most to develop on this notion that it is the client and not the therapist who knows best, because change is ultimately driven by actualizing forces within the person. It is to the work of Carl Rogers we now turn.

Carl Rogers and the actualizing tendency

As we have seen, Seligman in championing the ideas of positive psychology questioned the fundamental assumptions of mainstream psychology. Likewise, several decades before, Carl Rogers had questioned the fundamental assumptions of mainstream psychology in his day – dominated as it was then by Freudian ideas – proposing instead the view that human beings are organismically motivated towards developing to their full potential. As Rogers (1969) wrote:

> I have little sympathy with the rather prevalent concept that man is basically irrational, and thus his impulses, if not controlled, would lead to destruction of others and self. Man's behavior is exquisitely rational, moving with subtle and ordered complexity toward the goals his organism is endeavoring to achieve. (p. 29)

Here Rogers did not mean that people act in rational ways all of the time in the everyday sense of the term, as obviously they do not. No, what he was getting at is a more complex idea that if we were to understand deeply the motives for another person's behaviour we will see that they are doing their best organismically to be the most fully functioning they can. Even the most destructive behaviour is an expression, albeit a thwarted, usurped and distorted one, of an urge which is ultimately seeking to optimize the person's potential.

Deep within us, Rogers proposed, human beings are striving to become all that they can be. Rogers referred to this directional force of becoming as the actualizing tendency. In his important 1959 paper he wrote:

> This is the inherent tendency of the organism to develop all its capacities in ways which serve to maintain or enhance the organism. It involves not only the tendency to meet what Maslow terms 'deficiency needs' for air, food, water, and the like, but also more generalized activities. It involves development toward the differentiation of organs and of functions, expansion in terms of growth, expansion of effectiveness through the use of tools, expansion and enhancement through reproduction. It is development toward autonomy and away from heteronomy, or control by external forces. (p. 196)

Rogers (1959) conceptualized the basic directionality of the actualizing tendency as being toward the development of autonomous determination, expansion and effectiveness, and constructive social behaviour. The actualizing tendency, Rogers argued, was the one natural motivational force of human beings and which is always directed towards constructive growth. Later he added:

> It is the urge which is evident in all organic and human life – to expand, extend, to become autonomous, develop, mature – the tendency to express and activate all the capacities of the organism, to the extent that such activation enhances the organism or the self. (Rogers, 1961, p. 35)

To vividly illustrate the concept, Rogers (1961) described how during a vacation he was overlooking one of the rugged coves which dot the coastline of northern California:

> Several large rock outcroppings were at the mouth of the cove, and these received the full force of the great pacific combers which, beating upon them, broke into mountains of spray before surging into the cliff-lined shore. As I watched the waves breaking over these large rocks in the distance, I noticed with surprise what appeared to be tiny palm trees on the rocks, no more than two or three feet high, taking the pounding of the breakers. Through my binoculars I saw that these were some type of seaweed, with a slender 'trunk' topped off with a head of leaves. As one examined a specimen in the intervals between the waves it seemed clear that this fragile, erect, top-heavy plant would be utterly crushed and broken by the next breaker. When the wave crunched down upon it, the trunk bent almost flat, the leaves were whipped

into a straight line by the torrent of water, yet the moment the wave had passed, here was the plant again, erect, tough, resiliant. . . . Here in this palm-like seaweed was the tenacity of life, the forward thrust of life, the ability to push into an incredibly hostile environment and not only hold its own, but to adapt, develop, and become itself. (pp. 1–2)

Rogers used this example of how all organisms, be they palmlike seaweed or people, can be counted on to be directed toward maintaining, enhancing and reproducing. For Rogers, the actualizing tendency was thought to be the basic and sole motivation of people – a universal motivation always resulting in growth, development and auton-omy of the individual. In writing about the actualizing tendency, Rogers (1963a) states:

We are, in short, dealing with an organism which is always motivated, is always 'up to something', always seeking. So I would reaffirm, perhaps even more strongly after the passage of a decade, my belief that there is one central source of energy in the human organism; that it is a function of the whole organism rather than some portion of it; and that it is best conceptualized as a tendency toward fulfilment, toward actualization, toward the maintenance and enhancement of the organism. (p. 6)

This idea of the tendency towards actualization is, I would argue, one of the 'big ideas' of psychology. Other well-known theorists in the history of psychology who have pro-posed some form of actualizing tendency also include Adler (1927), Angyal (1941), Goldstein (1939), Jung (1933), Maslow (1968) and Rank (1936). As such it is an idea with a distinguished heritage. But it has been a controversial concept in contemporary mainstream psychology (see Ryan, 1995) and largely forgotten about, at least until the advent of positive psychology and its challenge to reflect on the philosophical roots of psychological practice (Nafstad, 2015). Within positive psychology the idea of the meta-theory of a tendency towards actualization is however gaining ground as a para-digm but traced back to the writings of Aristotle (Nafstad, 2015).

There is also much resonance in this idea with ideas from the East. As Hansard (2001) writes in his popular book on *The Tibetan Art of Living*:

The seeds within the fruit only know one thing: that they must grow, blossom and bear fruit. Essentially, we human beings must do the same, but some of us have forgotten. The truth is everywhere, in all things, in all situations and is behind the beginning and completion of everything. It can lead you to your spiritual potential and, most of all, it can reveal to you how to live your own life. (p. 19)

Foundation of the person-centred approach

The idea of the tendency towards actualization is the foundation of the person-centred therapeutic approach to therapy (e.g., Bohart, 2013; Joseph & Patterson, 2008; Mearns, Thorne, & McLeod, 2013). As I shall go on to discuss throughout this book, the implication of this big idea for professional psychological practice that the client knows best and can be trusted to find their own directions in life.

A common rejoinder to this might be, 'well if the client knows best what are they coming to therapy for?' But this is to misunderstand the idea of the client knowing best. It is not that people can easily articulate their best directions in life. It is a more complex notion that as organisms we have felt sense of what is right for us, as colloquially expressed in the idea of knowing in one's gut. Person-centred therapy therefore is a way for people to get in touch with their inner voice.

In short, it is the idea that people have the resources within them to know best what is right for themselves, and if they have the right support people can begin to access those resources for themselves so as to be able to determine their own solutions and directions. By the right support what this refers to is feeling sufficiently valued, understood and respected, with no expectations to be other than true to oneself. Under these conditions one's defences dissolve allowing one to confront oneself openly and honestly, allowing expression of the tendency towards actualization, towards becoming more fully functioning.

Joseph and Murphy (2013b) have conceptualized person-centred practice as at the centre of a Venn-diagram consisting of three overlapping circles representing: 1) the meta-theory of the tendency towards actualization, 2) relational ways of helping and 3) positive psychology with its emphasis on optimal functioning (see Figure 3.1).

In this way, we can consider person-centred therapy as being at the centre of these three overlapping circles. It is a relationship-based approach grounded in the meta-theoretical approach that people are intrinsically motivated towards optimal positive psychological functioning.

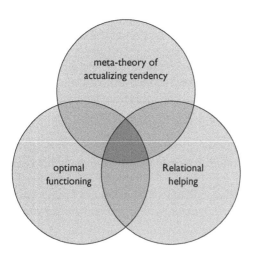

Figure 3.1 Venn diagram showing that person-centred therapy is located at the interface of the theory of actualization, positive psychology and relational helping.

Other forms of psychotherapy and counselling may also be relational or orientated towards positive functioning but what makes person-centred therapy unique is its combination of these and its grounding in the meta-theory of a tendency towards actualization.

In light of this Venn-diagram it may be helpful to go back to the previous chapter and to consider how each of the therapies described as positive psychotherapies sit within this structure in terms of their fundamental assumptions, relational focus and positive orientation.

As already mentioned, the implication of the person-centred approach is that people are their own best experts. It is worth now examining in more detail exactly why this is such a radical idea in practice.

The client as their own best expert

Rogers emphasized that it was how the individual perceives reality that was important and that the best vantage point for understanding a person is that person. In this respect Rogers' ideas resonate well with the ideas of cognitive therapy. However, although cognitive therapy also emphasizes that it is how the person perceives reality that is important, cognitive therapy does not necessarily adopt the view that it is the client who knows best what direction to go in. The majority of cognitive therapists adopt the view that they are able to show the client a different way to look at their situation, to teach new ways of thinking, on the basis of the assumption that people need some direction from the therapist.

Insofar as therapy is akin to the practice of medicine this idea is not strange. After all, if we break our leg we do need help from someone who is more expert than us to help us to know what to do. But Rogers' approach was a challenge to the idea that therapy was akin to the practice of medicine. Instead, as we have seen, his approach was about facilitating a person's ability to listen to their own inner wisdom and to be their own best expert because he believed in the tendency towards actualization as the single underlying motivational force.

How has the idea of therapy as being akin to medicine come to dominate the professional practice? There are a variety of possible reasons for this. One reason can be clearly traced from the early history of clinical psychology (Maddux, Snyder, & Lopez, 2004). Early clinical psychology training took place in psychiatric hospitals and clinics under the supervision of psychiatrists who were trained in medicine and psychoanalysis, thus permeating the fledgling profession of clinical psychology with the illness ideology and the medical model. Subsequently, in the United States, the establishment of the Veterans Administration after the Second World War created training centres and standards for clinical psychologists, but these were again steeped in the tradition of psychiatrists. Further, the founding of the United States National Institute of Mental Health channelled millions of research dollars toward the understanding and treatment of mental illness, thus further influencing the direction in which clinical psychology evolved (Maddux et al., 2004). These developments allowed a rise in status for the profession of clinical psychology, but one which required its adoption of the illness ideology and the medical model, so as to maintain consistency with its psychiatric masters (Maddux et al., 2004).

I believe that the medical model and the illness ideology are simply the wrong way to think about psychological suffering. By recognizing the client as the expert in their own life the person-centred therapist has a commitment not to be the expert over the other person and not to impose on clients the expert power given to them by social norms. As Brazier (1993) said:

> The bedrock of Rogers' philosophy was the notion that the person is a living experiencing organism whose basic tendencies are trustworthy. It is still difficult for most people in the modern age to appreciate how revolutionary this simple idea is. It is not until we start to consider how much of our energy in modern society is spent on building and maintaining structures, the primary purpose of which is to eliminate the (dangerous) human element from human interactions, that we begin to get a glimpse of how radical Rogers' vision was and still is. (pp. 7–8)

In recent years, it is encouraging that many new voices are joining this protest. Some of these voices even belong to clinical psychologists and psychiatrists. Person-centred theorists argue that those who adopt the medical model and the illness ideology damage their clients, and impede their potential for optimal functioning (see Sanders, 2005).

However, while change appears to be beginning to take place, the medical model is still widely accepted among the psychological professions and it will take some time to extricate the profession of psychology and reorient it towards a more productive framework for understanding psychological suffering and well-being.

In summary, the implication of the notion of the tendency towards actualization is that the client is their own best expert. Consequently, one rejects the medical model view in which it is the therapist whose expertise directs the course of the therapy. As such, the therapist needs to be able to go with the flow of the client.

Consider the following illustrative example. One client, John, a man in his early forties, came into therapy seeking help with his self-confidence at work, saying that his lack of confidence, for example, when it came to speaking up in meetings, was holding him back in his career. During therapy, he also began to discuss what he disliked about his job, and came to the realization that although he had a potentially rewarding career ahead of him financially, it was not a career that gave him a sense of purpose or joy in his life. He simply did not enjoy his work. It was a career he had fallen into after leaving university. At university he had studied management and accountancy, subjects that had not really interested him but which he had chosen following the advice of his parents. He had always wanted to write, and would have liked to study writing or literature at university, and wondered what his life would have been like if he had chosen this path instead. Over time, John began to develop his self-confidence, but also he became more interested in exploring these other issues, and he began to turn his attention to using his skills in this new direction, enrolling in an evening class on writing, and beginning to work on his writing ideas, submitting one of his stories to a competition. As the therapy progressed it was no longer used by John to develop his existing career but to find a way to exit his existing career and seek new opportunities and a way of living his life that felt more authentic.

As this example demonstrates, the person-centred approach rests on the idea that the agenda for change comes from the client rather than from the therapist. John's agenda was initially focused on developing his self-confidence in order to progress his career, but over time in therapy he introduced other issues, to do with his earlier choices in life, and with his aspirations to be a writer. The therapist's agenda was to stay with John's frame of reference and to explore those issues raised by John himself. In private practice this was not an issue for the therapist, and it was seen as a mark of success by John that he had begun to 'find himself'.

Reflections on human nature

Therapists have many choices as to how to respond to what a person tells them. They can give advice, ask questions, make diagnoses, reassure, listen, administer tests or interpret, to name but a few of the responses that might assist the person to make changes in their life. A new client arrives and sits down in the chair opposite us. What does the therapist do next? Jaqui tells us about a humiliating experience at work and bursts into laughter as she recounts the story. Another client, Frances, tells us about abusive experiences in childhood in a cold and matter-of-fact-way. Yet another client, Jennifer, with tears streaming from her eyes, says how unhappy and trapped she feels in her marriage. How ought a therapist to respond to each of these clients? Should we laugh with our client if we also find their story funny? Should we let our client know how we hear them being so 'matter-of-fact' despite what were clearly very emotionally distressing experiences? Should we let our client know how sad we feel to hear their story?

As a teacher of counselling and psychotherapy I often meet with students who are confused about how to 'do' therapy. Is it okay to ask questions? Should I answer questions that the client asks me? Can I say what I think? Answers to these questions depend on our view of what therapy is and what we think we are doing. As I have said, to me the most practical thing one can do as a new therapist, or indeed even as an experienced therapist, is to consider deeply one's ideas about human nature.

Our ideas about human nature are at the core of how we practise as therapists. It is probably true to say that questions about human nature did not figure as highly in mainstream psychology until positive psychology came along and challenged the status quo. But such considerations were always at the core of Rogers' views on therapy.

To Rogers, therapy was the meeting of two people. It is the depth of relationship that forms between them that is important. Although informed by science, the practice of therapy is an art – an expression of our ability to relate with another person at the deepest levels, and to be able to confront the existential truths that face us all, in a way that is sometimes humorous, often creative and always fully human. What the evidence tells us, time and again, is the importance of the relationship between therapist and client (see Bozarth & Motomasa, 2005).

Scientific findings can tell us about the associations between various cognitive and emotional factors, between therapeutic interventions and psychological outcomes, but scientific results are not able to tell us how we ought to interact with other people in the application of that science. In an influential paper, Brodley (2005a) argued that psychotherapy is limited as a scientific activity because whether we are conscious of it or not, psychotherapy is always an expression of our values and attitudes.

The practice of therapy is an art. As Wampold (2001) put it so well:

> The performer's grounding in music theory is invisible to the audience unless the canons of composition are violated in such a way as the performance is discordant. Similarly, the master therapist, informed by psychological knowledge and theory and guided by experience, produces an artistry that assists clients to move ahead in their lives with meaning and health. (p. 225)

It is important to understand the process of therapy intellectually, but that in itself does not make for effective practice. Similarly, it is important to be able to relate to others, but that too, in itself, does not make for effective practice as a therapist. Artistry arises through the skilful application of theory. What I will now go on to argue is that how we decide upon our artistry depends ultimately on our fundamental theoretical assumptions about human nature.

The need to reflect on our ontological position is not a novel idea, since all experienced therapists understand that there are different therapeutic schools, all of which are founded upon basic assumptions about human nature (see Joseph, 2010 for a review of the therapeutic models). However, mainstream professional psychology approaches have become so entrenched within the medical model that it is easy to lose sight of the fact that what one does is founded upon basic and very deep-seated assumptions about human nature. The following section is intended as a prompt for discussion in classroom situations.

Each of us has deep-seated beliefs about human nature. For example, some people believe that God created us all and that human nature is divine whereas others believe that we are the products of evolutionary forces and human nature is instinctual. Whatever the truth is on this issue, the fact is that different people believe different things, and what people believe has a profound influence on how they choose to live their lives (see Table 3.1).

Everyone has their own way of looking at the world. There are many conflicting views on human nature, with many religious leaders, scientists, philosophers and psychologists all holding different views on human nature. Our beliefs about human nature are so deep-seated that we rarely question them, and yet they fundamentally influence our attitude towards people and our understandings of why

Table 3.1 Exercise: Exploring your views about human nature

Here are some statements about human nature. Read each one and respond quickly as to whether you think it is true or false. Don't think too hard about your answer, give your instant reaction, just respond as quickly as you can, and let your heart say yes or no to each of the following statements.

People are basically generous.

People are basically selfish.

People are basically greedy.

People are basically kind.

People are basically loving.

People are basically bad.

The immediate reaction of some people on reading those three statements is true, false, false, false, true, true, and false. For other people, their gut reaction is false, true, true, false, false, true. Other people have a more mixed response, but essentially people fall into one of two categories on reading those statements, either they have what might be characterized as a positive view of human nature, or they have what might be characterized as a negative view of human nature. Your gut reaction to those statements will possibly tell you something about your own philosophy of human nature, whether you have a basically negative or positive view of human nature.

people do the things that they do. As therapists, our fundamental assumptions underpin the very way in which we choose to work with people. As such, they are of pervasive importance to our therapeutic practice. Try the exercise in Table 3.2 as a starting point for reflection on your own views why people behave as they do.

This issue is especially important for trainee psychologists and other novice therapists, whose training equips them to use a variety of different techniques, but often without reflection on their basic assumptions. To practise as a therapist we must surely hold that people have the capacity for change? That is a first and obvious assumption.

But then we must reflect on our assumptions about how change is possible. This is not so obvious. The deep-seated assumptions of a therapist are seen in their choice of words. When asked about their practice, one therapist will talk about getting the client to 'move on', another will talk about their task being to 'understand the client's history', yet another will talk about their 'management of the client's symptoms'. Each is giving a taste of his or her own views of human nature, and about how those views of human nature fundamentally influence them in their practice of striving to help another person.

In those contexts where all share similar views, the deep-seated assumptions go unnoticed because there are no points of contrast. If, for example, in the seminar room everyone is talking about getting the client to move on, no one notices that this is a way of talking that announces the meaning system of those in the

Table 3.2 Exploring your perceptions of why people behave as they do

The following exercise can be carried out in groups and used to form the basis of discussion to explore differences in perception.

Now read the following question and then answer whether you think the answer is A, B, or C.

1   When people are selfish, greedy, or unkind is it mostly because . . . ?

    A   of the way they were brought up.
    B   they were just born that way.
    C   of the circumstances in which they are living.

2   When people are loving, kind, and generous, is it mostly because . . . ?

    A   of the way they were brought up.
    B   they were just born that way.
    C   of the circumstances in which they are living.

room. When a therapist talks about getting their client to 'move on', there is the message that it is the therapist who knows what the client needs to do next. When a therapist talks about the need to understand the client's history, there is the message that this is important and useful in order to help the client. When a therapist talks about the management of 'symptoms', there is the message that the client's problems are symptomatic of some psychological disorder.

The point of these examples above is to emphasize that any practice of psychotherapy rests on the therapist's fundamental assumptions about human nature. These assumptions are easily heard in our choice of words. Therapists' assumptions reflect their personalities and preferences, forged through their life experiences and therapeutic training. These assumptions may be uncritically accepted by practitioners trained in a particular model and a particular way of working and simply taken for granted and unchallenged, assuming the position of the status quo.

The challenge of the person-centred approach is to consider the implication of the notion that people possess a tendency towards actualization. Person-centred theorists consider the implications to be that therapists should go at the client's pace and direction, so in that sense they are not getting them to move on; that they will willingly explore with their client his or her personal history, but only if that is what the client has brought along, not because they think this is what ought to be done; and that they will not introduce the notion of symptoms because the person-centred therapist does not accept the idea that the person is ill.

The heart of the person-centred approach is simply the act of respecting the other person's right to self-determination. This is more complicated than it sounds because to respect someone's right to self-determination you have to do so for its own sake because it is the ethical thing to do, not because it achieves another desired goal. If I respect your right to self-determination because my goal is to make you do something other than what you are doing, then by definition I'm not actually respecting your right to self-determination. Rather, I am trying to make you change in a way that I think you ought to. In a sense I am only pretending to you and to myself that I respect your right to self-determination.

For this reason, the person-centred therapist's agenda is to genuinely respect the client's self-determination, with the understanding that it is when people experience themselves as self-determining agents that they will make the best decisions for themselves that they can, and that as a result the client will move in the direction of becoming more fully functioning, whatever that looks like for that person. As such the person-centred therapist has no agenda that the client should change in any particular way, or even at all.

Conclusion

Positive psychology provided the impetus to re-examine our fundamental assumptions about human nature, particularly with regard to the medical model. The ideas of Carl Rogers about the actualizing tendency as the core motivational force for optimal human development promises to provide an alternative to the illness ideology. In this chapter, I have discussed what I see as some fundamental issues for the practice of positive therapy. These issues challenge us as psychologists and as practitioners to be reflective of the way we work with people and, equally importantly, of the 'why' we work with people in the way we do. Fundamental assumptions about human nature can be broadly grouped into three positions: that people are by nature intrinsically motivated by destructive impulses that need to be controlled; that people are blank slates upon which either motivations for destructive or constructive impulses may be written, or that people are by nature intrinsically motivated by positive, constructive directional tendencies towards the actualization of their potentialities.

We also saw that the person-centred approach offers a genuinely positive psychological perspective. By definition, person-centred psychology with its emphasis on becoming fully functioning is a positive psychology. But in contrast, positive psychology is not necessarily person-centred unless it adopts the meta-theoretical principle of a universal actualizing tendency.

In conclusion for this chapter, it is not what the therapist *does* (i.e., their technique) that determines whether a therapy is person-centred. Rather it is what the therapist *thinks* (i.e. their fundamental assumptions), that is important. The crux of being a person-centred therapist is that the therapist adopts a way of thinking which embraces the notion that their task is to facilitate the client's actualizing tendency. It is not a form of therapy that appeals to everyone. Some readers may disagree strongly with the person-centred approach to human nature, in which case it is not for them. Nonetheless, it is our ideas about human nature that make us the psychotherapists we are. We cannot avoid fundamental assumptions – all therapies are ultimately based on some notion or other of what it is to be human – so the question is which assumptions will guide what you do.

Further reading

Rogers, C. R. (1961). *On becoming a person*. Boston, MA: Houghton Mifflin.
One of Rogers' books in which he presents his ideas in an engaging way with the hindsight of over two decades' work behind him.

Rogers, C. R. (1963a). The actualizing tendency in relation to 'motives' and to consciousness. In M. Jones (ed.), *Nebraska symposium on motivation, Vol 11* (pp. 1–24). Lincoln: University of Nebraska Press.
A more detailed treatise on the actualizing tendency.

Joseph, S., & Murphy, D. (2013b). Person-centered approach, positive psychology and relational helping: Building bridges. *Journal of Humanistic Psychology, 53*, 26–51.
Our paper in the *Journal of Humanistic Psychology* in which we first discuss the three overlapping circles.

Chapter 4

Developmental and personality theory

In the previous chapter I introduced the notion of the actualizing tendency as the theoretical foundation for a positive psychology of psychotherapy. As we have seen, this is a somewhat revolutionary idea as it implies that people can trust themselves to know their own best directions in life. Thus, the task of the therapist is to help the person to listen to their own inner voice of wisdom. In this chapter, I will elaborate further on person-centred theory and its main concepts – need for positive regard, conditional and unconditional positive regard, self-concept, self-structure, conditions of worth, the organismic valuing process, and fully functioning. Then I will examine contemporary positive psychology theory and research, showing how it is consistent with person-centred theory.

A theory of therapy, personality, and interpersonal relationships

The theoretical background to the person-centred approach was published by Rogers (1959) in his chapter 'A theory of therapy, personality, and interpersonal relationships, as developed in the client-centred framework' which appeared in Koch's *Psychology: A Study of a Science*. It is a theory of human development and personality.

Remembering the metaphor from Yalom in the previous chapter about how an acorn becomes an oak, right from the outset of life the newborn infant strives to become what it has the potential to be. As the infant gurgles and grasps and is bombarded by the stimuli of the world around, the infant is not yet able to differentiate between 'me' and 'not me' experiences. As yet the infant has no view of itself. But over months and years as she explores the world she begins to make this differentiation between 'me' and 'not me' experiences, and the *self-concept* begins to emerge. This process is described as *self-actualization*.[1]

Organismic valuing process

Initially, self-actualization is driven by the *organismic valuing process* (OVP). The OVP refers to the process intrinsic to the organism by which it continually evaluates experiences in relation to the actualizing tendency. It implies that human organisms can be relied on through their physiological processes to know what they need from their environment and what is right for them for the self-actualization of their potentialities. Through the OVP people come to develop a self-concept based on their evaluation of experiences. However, as the self-concept emerges so too does the child's awareness of others and their *need for positive regard*.

Need for positive regard

Rogers' argument was that the need for positive regard, or to be loved, was a universal need that was pervasive and persistent. Human beings need contact with others (Warner, 2002). Contemporary evolutionary psychologists would hold with this notion as well because it makes sense that we need to build bonds and a sense of belonging with those around us if we are to survive.

When the two processes of the need for positive regard and the OVP are in harmony, or congruent, then the child continues to move towards becoming *fully functioning*. However, positive regard from others comes in two forms, conditional and unconditional.

Whereas *unconditional positive regard* allows the universal motivational force towards growth and development within us, free rein, such that we move towards satisfying our needs for autonomy and belonging, this directional developmental force becomes thwarted by *conditional positive regard.*

The smiling infant guided by OVP reaches out to her parent but in doing so knocks over a drink that the parent has. Luckily she is not hurt but the parent reacts in shock and pushes the infant away towards safety. The parents are over-anxious and fearful for the safety of their child. The infant is confused and interprets this experience in her limited age-related way – perhaps that she should not seek attention or reach out towards her parents. This is one minor event in a series of hundreds of thousands yet to come that will all be part of the developmental experiences that shape how she understands herself in the world. A few years later Jill falls from a swing and runs crying to her parents with a graze on her knee. Her father, preoccupied at that moment with his own worries about an event in his workplace, turns to her and says for her not to be such a cry baby. Feeling scolded, she stops crying and runs away to hide. It is through this process that *conditions of worth* develop.

Conditions of worth

OVP guides us towards seeking environments that are conducive to our development. However, OVP becomes easily thwarted and usurped by *conditions of worth* that are introjected from external sources. The term introjected refers to how these conditions begin as external to us but how, over time, we internalize them as our own, such that we become estranged from our organismic needs. There is a loss of ability to trust the evidence of one's own senses, accompanied by the emergence of a tendency to defer to the judgement of others in order to determine the value of an experience. Jill, for example, has learned that it is best to hide emotions from others and it is from this point of view that she evaluates her experiences.

In this respect she has become alienated from the actualization tendency, lost the ability to trust the evidence of her own senses and her OVP. Instead she defers to her introjected condition of worth that holds that emotions are to be avoided. She begins to develop ways of processing emotional material that are dysfunctional.

It is through the above developmental process that the self-structure is shaped. The self-structure refers to the overall personality structure and includes the self-concept. For most people, by the time they reach adolescence they are alienated from themselves to varying degrees in the sense of being out of touch with their OVP and their self-structure contains a variety of defensive processes.

As such, whereas the tendency towards actualization was posited by Rogers to be positive and prosocial, self-actualization is not, it simply refers to how the self is realized through the dual process of the tension that exists between the OVP and conditions of worth.

Imagine a few years later, Jill is now a timid girl, uncertain of herself and her place in the world. Jill has now started school. Her parents are worried about her. She interprets from her parents the message that to be loved, she must do well at school. This is not to say that the parents intend harm to their child, but they are anxious and fearful for her future. As such they want her to do well at school knowing that this will give her more choices later on in life. But the child has a need to feel loved and valued, and she quickly learns that to receive love from her parents, she must do well at school. She comes home with a glowing report card and receives warm loving praise from her parents. As a child wanting to be loved and valued she comes to learn that this is what she must do. 'To be loved I must do well'. The child introjects this message, that to be loved one must succeed in life, which is said to be a *condition of worth* for her. She grows up learning to value herself only to the extent that she does well at school, and later, that she does well in her career. It is hard for her. She struggles through school. Her self-regard suffers as her grades are not as good as she knows they should be. But she keeps her feelings to herself. No one knows how unhappy she is. If asked, her parents would say she was a bright and happy girl who enjoyed school.

Many years later, Jill has become an adult, her parents have passed away, and she no longer needs to do well at school (or in her career) in order to please them. However, the message to succeed is so deeply internalized in the psyche of the woman that she accepts it as part of herself. The motivational force to actualize has been thwarted and usurped in pursuit of the need to achieve well in her career, and rather than listening to her own inner voice, she is, so to speak, still listening to the voice of her parents that she had introjected in childhood. She has worked hard and is a solicitor in a leading firm. Her hours are long and that suits her.

Often people cannot articulate easily what their conditions of worth are, so deeply buried are they within them. As the above example demonstrates, conditions of worth are often very subtle. Nevertheless, this subtlety is all the more powerful, since it can render us unaware of what our conditions of worth are, with the influence being much more subtle and lasting far longer than might ostensibly appear to be the case.

Central to the theory is the assumption that we have a need to be positively regarded, and will seek regard from our social environment. If all that is on offer is conditional regard, then that is what we reach out for. For most of us, we grow up with a mix of unconditional and conditional regard from the world around us. We are surrounded by conditions of worth, which we receive from our parents or other carers, teachers and religious educators, media, television and so on. All of these messages tell us about what is important in life, and what we must do to be valued. All of us introject conditions of worth, and to varying extents self-actualize in the direction of our conditions of worth, rather than how we would have self-actualized if we had received only unconditional positive regard.

None of us are fully able to escape the influences of the world around us. Whereas the theory of the tension between the actualizing tendency and conditions of worth is universal, the specific nature of that tension is unique to each of us. In the same way that each acorn has the potential to be the best oak tree it can be, no two acorns, becoming shoots and then saplings, receive the exact same environments. No two oak trees are identical. Some people's conditions of worth are held so strongly that their actualizing tendency has become so thwarted and usurped, so that they self-actualize in a direction wholly consistent with their conditions of worth as opposed to the actualizing tendency.

In this way, when self-actualization is incongruent with the actualizing tendency, then problems in living arise. As in the example above, Jill's conditions of worth were to do well at school. She learned to work hard at school to please her parents because to do otherwise she believed would result in the loss of their positive regard. This is not to say that Jill was aware that this is what she was doing. Throughout her adult life Jill had tried to live to these values that she had internalized in childhood, and although successful in her career her satisfaction with life was low, and she was often irritable with those around her, and depressed in her mood. It was through her diagnosis of depression that she entered counselling through which she began to realize that she did not actually enjoy her work. As she began to listen more closely to herself she began to realize that deep within herself the values she was living were not hers but those of her parents, or at least the messages that she had introjected as a young girl about what was important. The things that mattered to her she had left behind long ago in childhood, her freedom of expression and creativity, in preference for the things that seemed to matter to other people.

Reflections on conditions of worth

Each of us has our own conditions of worth, to work hard, to please others, to be strong – imagine, if love is withheld from a child when she cries, she gets the message 'in order to be loved, I mustn't cry' (see Table 4.1).

It is empowering to understand our own conditions of worth. A simple exercise to help do this is presented in Table 4.2. Of course, the exercise will be used differently by different people as not everyone will have had both parents available to them. As such, therapists would of course vary the exercise appropriately for the person they were with. The exercise can also be used as part of a group

Table 4.1 Example conditions of worth

- To be successful
- To please others
- To bottle up emotions
- To defer to authority
- To not get angry
- To be grateful for what you have
- To not make a fuss

Table 4.2 Exploring our own conditions of worth

First, it is necessary to get into a state of relaxation.

Then, with your eyes closed, imagine going back in time to the house of your childhood. Imagine the younger you standing there at the front door of the house of your childhood. Now go in, walk into your house, now imagine seeing your father, picture him standing there, he turns towards you, and he says to you, 'whatever you do in life, you must always. . . . ' Now finish the sentence. You must always . . . what? Don't think too hard, just say to yourself whatever comes immediately to mind.

Now imagine seeing your mother, picture her standing there, she turns to you and says, 'whatever you do in life, you must always . . . ' Finish the sentence. You must always . . . what?

The exercise is used to reflect upon how early experiences with your caregivers affected how you are today. The sort of things that people finish these sentences with are things like:

     . . . work hard to get what you want

     . . . be nice to people if you don't want them to be cross with you

     . . . listen to what other people tell you to do

     . . . do as you are told

     . . . wash your hands before dinner

     . . . say your prayers if you want God to love you

     . . . say thank you for what you've got

     . . . try hard even if it's not good enough

     . . . be good

     . . . hit people back

     . . . hide your tears

     . . . be strong

     . . . love your parents no matter what

     . . . remember that I love you no matter what

In thinking about the above exercise you might have had some sentence completions of your own come to mind. They might be similar to some of the ones listed, or ones that are unique to you. People are often surprised by what this exercise reveals to them, it can be a very powerful exercise in helping people to understand their own conditions of worth.

teaching exercise and trainees may find it useful to work in small groups allowing them to discuss their conditions of worth, and to share their experiences.

What is important is for the person to think about the people who were very significant to them when they were growing up, to open up to the deep-seated messages they carry within them about what is important in life. The exercise is used to reflect upon how early experiences with your caregivers affected how you are today. Sometimes this can be a very upsetting exercise too and therapists need to be cautious in their use of such exercises.

It is essential as a person-centred therapist to be knowledgeable about one's own conditions of worth and how these influence our choices in life and our work with clients. The person-centred therapist strives to live a life free from conditions of worth. It may also be helpful to consider how your own conditions of worth influence your choices in life.

In summary, conditions of worth are those messages we introject from society and those around us about how we should behave if we are to be accepted and valued. As a consequence we learn to distort and deny certain experiences so that they fit with our picture of self, and we self-actualize in a way consistent with our conditions of worth rather than our actualizing tendency. Thus, the theory dictates that in a social environment characterized by conditional positive regard, people will self-actualize not in a direction consistent with their actualizing tendency, but in a direction consistent with their conditions of worth. As Rogers (1959) said:

> This, as we see it, is the basic estrangement in man. He has not been true to himself, to his natural organismic valuing of experience, but for the sake of preserving the positive regard of others has now come to falsify some of the values he experiences and to perceiving them in terms based only on their value to others. Yet this has not been a conscious choice, but a natural – and tragic – development in infancy. (p. 226)

We will return to how conditions of worth are the basis for estrangement later in Chapter 7 when we consider person-centred psychopathology, but for the moment I want to return us to the other side of the coin, and how person-centred theory is a positive psychology.

What the theory says is that when the social environment is characterized by *unconditional positive regard*, the child is able to learn that he or she is valued with no strings attached. Thus, rather than learn to listen to others about what they have to do to get love, they learn to listen to themselves. They do not introject beliefs about how they should be, but come to regard themselves unconditionally.

Unconditional positive self-regard

The concept of unconditional positive self-regard is central to person-centred therapy. As we have seen the person-centred approach is a developmental theory that proposes that we have a basic and universal need for positive regard from others. The infant learns to respond in ways that result in receiving love and affection from parents, caregivers and significant others. However, as love and affection from others can be communicated either conditionally or unconditionally the child's positive self-regard can take these two forms (Rogers, 1959). Unconditional positive self-regard refers to a person's acceptance of all of his or her subjective experiences, without reference to the perceived attitudes, rules or values of others, in such a way that they relate to themselves with warmth, compassion and a non-judgemental understanding.

Thus, *Unconditional positive self-regard* refers to the individual's acceptance of all of his or her subjective experiences, without reference to either the perceived attitudes of others or to rules or values that have been internalized from the social environment. It involves relating to all of one's experiences, whether positive or negative, with warmth and a non-judgemental understanding. People differ in the extent to which they unconditionally regard themselves.

Unconditional positive self-regard therefore allows the self-actualization of the person and the actualizing tendency to be co-ordinated, such that there is a 'unitary actualizing tendency' (Rogers, 1963a, p. 20) (see Ford, 1991). In this way, the person self-actualizes to the fullest of their potential in ways that maximize their ability to be fully functioning.

Fully functioning

Rogers (1959) held that in a social environment characterized by unconditional positive regard, people will develop unconditional positive self-regard, and thus, unhindered by defences and distortions, will self-actualize in a direction consistent with their actualizing tendency towards becoming what he referred to as fully functioning human beings:

> 'The fully functioning person' is synonymous with optimal psychological adjustment, optimal psychological maturity, complete congruence, complete openness to experience . . . Since some of these terms sound somewhat static, as though such a person 'had arrived' it should be pointed out that all the characteristics of such a person are *process* characteristics. The fully functioning person would be a person-in-process, a person continually changing. (Rogers, 1959, p. 235; see also Rogers, 1963b)

The fully functioning person is someone who is accepting of themselves, values all aspects of themselves – their strengths and their weaknesses, is able to live fully in the present, experiences life as a process, finds purpose and meaning in life, desires authenticity in themselves, others, and societal organizations, values deep trusting relationships and is compassionate towards others, and able to receive compassion from others, and is acceptant that change is necessary and inevitable (see Merry, 1999) (see Table 4.3).

Table 4.3 Characteristics of the fully functioning person

Be open to experience.
Exhibit no defensiveness.
Be able to interpret experience accurately.
Have a flexible rather than static self-concept open to change through experience.
Trust in his or her own experiencing process and develop values in accordance with that experience.
Have no conditions of worth and experience unconditional self-regard.
Be able to respond to new experiences openly.
Be guided by his or her own valuing process through being fully aware of all experience, without the need for denial or distortion of any of it.
Be open to feedback from his or her environment and make realistic changes resulting from that feedback.
Live in harmony with others and experience the rewards of mutual positive regard.

The fully functioning person, however, is an ideal. Later, Rogers (1961) clarified this by describing how he saw 'The Good Life' as a process:

> It seems to me that the good life is not any fixed state. It is not, in my estimation, a state of virtue, or contentment, or nirvana, or happiness. It is not a condition in which the individual is adjusted, fulfilled, or actualized ... The good life is a *process*, not a state of being ... It is a direction, not a destination. The direction ... is that which is selected by the total organism, when there is psychological freedom to move in *any* direction. (pp. 186–187)

All of us have, to varying extents, self-actualized incongruently to our actualizing tendency. For some, incongruence is minimal, for others more substantial, and the more we struggle to hear our inner voice, the more we can be said to be in a state of incongruence. According to this view, the various psychological problems we may experience are manifestations of the internalization of conditions of worth.

In essence, what the theory is saying is that deep down each of us possesses an inner wisdom about how best to lead our lives. Each of us has a different best path to take in life, depending on our intrinsic characteristics, strengths and interests. Unfortunately, few people ever find themselves on exactly the right path for them. We all know people who would make a brilliant teacher, a compassionate doctor, a talented carpenter, an inspired artist, but who for one reason or another never found their path in life to take them there. The brilliant teacher instead works as a sales director, the compassionate doctor is a civil servant, the carpenter is a journalist, and the inspired artist works in marketing and advertising. They might be good at what they do, but each feels that what they do is 'just not them'. Of course, it is not just about our employment, but this is the major way in which we come to express ourselves and our unique talents in our culture.

Thus, most of us actualize only a fraction of our full potential. We grow up to develop an image of ourselves that we show to the world. We use psychological defences to stop us hearing the truth about this image. We do not want to hear evidence that we are not as clever, attractive, witty, handsome or liked, as we tell ourselves. For this reason, we do not really get to know ourselves properly. We hide from knowing ourselves because the pain of self-knowledge is too great.

In an unconditional and accepting social environment where we feel valued, however, we can begin to drop our defences and confront the truth about ourselves. That is the essence of person-centred therapy, which we will discuss in the next chapter. But for the moment, we will consider person-centred personality theory in light of positive psychology.

Building bridges between person-centred theory and positive psychology research

Before we turn to the contemporary scene, it is interesting to reflect on the history of the person-centred approach within the field of psychology. As already mentioned Rogers was a psychologist by profession and the person-centred approach was a development within mainstream psychology. The key theoretical developments in person-centred theory were published in well-regarded psychology journals and books (Rogers, 1957, 1959). As such, person-centred psychology was seen as being at the cutting edge of applied psychology and attracted empirical researchers to test its propositions. The evidence was supportive of the theory and the therapy although of course it would now be seen as limited by the standards of statistical and methodological sophistication used today.

Later in his career Rogers moved away from working in academic psychological settings. This was the time of the 1960s and 1970s. Humanistic psychology was flourishing and Rogers' interest shifted to other applications of the theory such as the encounter group movement, educational practice, new ways of living and human relations more generally. Rogers and his colleagues were not precious about their work and encouraged others to be involved. As the field of counselling began to develop many were attracted to the person-centred approach. As such the person-centred approach began to develop a strong practitioner following, but now with much less of a research focus. Many of those who were interested in research emphasized people's unique experiences and adopted phenomenological methods rather than the traditional scientific methods.

Within academic psychological settings of the 1970s, however, the cognitive-behavioural approach was gaining in popularity and attracting the interest of clinical research scientists. Academic psychologists were now developing their empirical scientific research into the new cognitive-behavioural methods of therapy. The research into cognitive-behavioural therapies blossomed, while that of person-centred therapy was left behind. However, it is critical to remember that the relative absence of research support did not imply that person-centred therapy was not effective – rather, it was a reflection of the fact that it was not being subject to the same amount of empirical scrutiny that cognitive-behavioural techniques were.

As the 1980s and 1990s progressed, person-centred theory began to be seen as a historical footnote in the development of psychology, with many of the new generation of psychologists having no experience of it or knowledge of the past research. Nevertheless, the person-centred approach remained popular among counsellors and continued to evolve as the field of counselling became more established in the 1990s and beyond.

Today, with hindsight, we can look back at over 50 years of scholarship in the person-centred approach and see the profundity and complexity of Rogers' thinking, and that of his colleagues in the first generation of person-centred scholars, and understand their impact (see Barrett-Lennard, 1998; Kirschenbaum, 2007). The person-centred movement helped to pioneer many of the developments that are now key to contemporary psychology. First, as we have already seen, the person-centred approach predated positive psychology by 50 years with its emphasis on fully functioning experiences and behaviour. Second, by the 1970s and 1980s many of those who became interested in the person-centred approach were turning to phenomenological research methods. At the time this was controversial but today qualitative methods have gained academic respectability largely due to the pioneering work of many of these early humanistic psychologists. Third, it is only relatively recently that the mainstream agenda of clinical psychology has begun to realign with the person-centred agenda to question the medical model, the terminology of disorder, and whether the search for specific treatments has overshadowed the far more important consideration of the therapeutic relationship.

Psychological foundations for humanistic therapy

Person-centred therapy, for the reasons described above, became detached from mainstream psychological research. It may therefore come as a surprise to many in the person-centred tradition that there is a vast resource of empirical research in the developmental, social and personality psychology tradition that is consistent with and supportive of person-centred theory and therapy that has been overlooked by person-centred scholars until recently (Cooper & Joseph, in press).

Recently, Cooper and Joseph (in press) have reviewed the psychological literature for three ways in which it supports humanistic therapy. First, they point to the vast resource of research on the beneficial effects of social support. For example, research testifies that greater well-being is associated with feeling connected to others, social participation, and perceiving oneself to have friends to rely on in a crisis. Furthermore, they review the literature showing that poor or absent interpersonal connections are associated with the presence of mental health difficulties.

Second, they review the literature on emotional expression and how disclosing one's feelings can be beneficial, as evidenced by experimental studies as well as survey-based correlational studies. It may be because this reduces physiological arousal, reducing preoccupation and self-focused attention, and through allowing people to process and make sense of their experiences.

Third, they review the evidence for the role of authenticity and how those who score higher on tests for authenticity are more satisfied with life, higher in self-esteem, less depressed and anxious, more alert and awake and also have less physical symptoms such as headaches, aches and pains.

So, although proponents of person-centred theory have not been as active in gathering empirical evidence as proponents of other therapeutic approaches, critics are wrong when they say that the person-centred approach lacks research evidence. There is a huge amount of evidence in support of person-centred theory but it is to be found in the journals of social and personality psychology, rather than the journals of counselling and psychotherapy. In particular, evidence is to be found in self-determination theory (SDT) pioneered by psychologists Edward Deci and Richard Ryan (1985; 2000). This theory is one of the most influential theories in mainstream positive psychology in recent years, with striking similarities to person-centred theory, and which is supported by a substantial research effort.

Self-determination theory

Self-determination theory (SDT) (Deci & Ryan, 1985; 1991; 2000; Ryan & Deci, 2000) provides a similar meta-theoretical perspective to person-centred personality theory. SDT has three elements:

> The first is that human beings are inherently proactive, that they have the potential to act on and master both the inner forces (viz. their drives and emotions) and the external (i.e. environmental) forces they encounter, rather than being passively controlled by those forces. . . .
>
> Second, human beings, as self-organizing systems, have an inherent tendency toward growth, development, and integrated functioning. . . .
>
> The third important philosophical assumption is that, although activity and optimal development are inherent to the human organism, these do not happen automatically. For people to actualize their inherent nature and potentials – that is, to be optimally active and to develop effectively – they require nutrients from the social environment. To the extent that they are denied the necessary support and nourishment by chaotic, controlling, or rejecting environments, there will be negative consequences for their activity and development. (Deci & Vansteenkiste, 2004, pp. 23–24)

Although SDT theorists trace the different lineage of their work to Harlow (1953) and White (1959), rather than directly to Rogers, as will be evident from the previous chapter these are the same meta-theoretical elements that also constitute Rogers' person-centred personality theory (Rogers, 1959). At the meta-theoretical level, SDT and person-centred theory are synonymous (Patterson and Joseph, 2007a; Sheldon, 2013). This is an exciting convergence of ideas from these two traditions of psychological thought.

Mainstream psychological practice, however, adopts the opposite position to these three elements with their agenda of therapist expertise and implicit assumption that motivation for development needs to be externally imposed on the person. As argued throughout this book these meta-theoretical elements promise to provide the foundation stone for positive psychology of psychotherapy. Similarly, Deci and Vansteenkiste (2004) write:

> Although positive psychology researchers are working to identify factors that enhance individuals' capacities, development, and well-being, only a few . . . fully embrace and utilize this critical meta-theoretical assumption for grounding their research or building their theoretical perspectives. (p. 24)

In response to the above comment, it is worth emphasizing that the entire tradition of person-centred therapy rests on this same meta-theoretical assumption. This is a synergy between two traditions of theory and practice that has until now gone largely unnoticed. It is important for person-centred practitioners to understand that what they do is in fact supported by the research tradition of SDT, and it is important for SDT theorists to realize that there is a therapeutic tradition that embraces the meta-theoretical assumption, with over 50 years of discussion on the implications for practice.

Positive psychologists such as Deci and Vansteenkiste (2004) and Ryan (1995) are in agreement that the organismic valuing process is either supported or undermined by the social environment. SDT posits thus three basic psychological needs – autonomy, competence and relatedness – and theorizes that fulfilment of these needs is essential for growth. The need for autonomy concerns the need to be able to act through choice and volition. The need for competence concerns the need to be effective in dealing with the environment. The need for relatedness concerns the need to connect with others.These are not conceptualized as learned needs, but as an inherent aspect of human nature that can be seen across gender, across time and across culture (Chirkov, Ryan, Kim, & Kaplan, 2003). Deci and Vansteenkiste (2004) and Ryan (1995) have emphasized how the social environment must provide the nutrients for individuals' needs for autonomy, relatedness and competence. People are intrinsically motivated to move towards social environments that provide these needs.

SDT therefore defines the nutrients that the social environment must provide for intrinsic motivation to take place. Deci and Ryan (2000) agree that the social environment does not always meet these needs, and that when these needs are not met development is thwarted, leading to ill-being and alienation.

At first glance it may seem that SDT is proposing different factors than Rogers, who, as already discussed, emphasized the universal need people have for unconditional positive regard (UPR). But, when examined more closely it becomes clear that these differences between Deci and Ryan's conceptualization of need satisfactions and Rogers' conceptualization of UPR are not that different from each other. In fact, I would say that they are essentially describing the opposite sides of the same coin. Unconditionality is the way to support autonomy. Positive regard is the way to support relatedness.

We can see the similarities if we look at how Deci and Ryan, and their colleagues have measured the concept of needs satisfaction. For example, in one study by La Guardia, Ryan, Couchman, & Deci (2000) of parental influence, a questionnaire was developed that asked respondents to rate items measuring needs satisfactions. Inspection of items used to measure autonomy (e.g. *my mother allows me to decide things for myself*), competence (e.g. *my mother puts time and energy into helping me*), and relatedness (e.g. *my mother accepts me and likes me as I am*), could equally well be conceptualized as measuring the broader concept of unconditional positive regard: i.e. unconditionality (*my mother allows me to decide things for myself*), and positive regard (*my mother accepts me and likes me as I am*). The difference between unconditional positive regard and need satisfactions is simply terminological.

As I see it, the point of UPR, expressed in the language of SDT, is to support both the autonomy and relatedness needs of the person in the understanding that their competence subsequently develops. In Rogers (1959) definition of the actualizing tendency, the organism is intrinsically motivated towards autonomy, competence and relatedness. Thus, Rogers and Deci and Ryan provide broadly similar accounts of the same processes. SDT and person-centred theory obviously share much common ground and we are left with some interesting questions for future research and theoretical discussion. For example, does an unconditional positively regarding social environment as posited by Rogers (1957; 1959) sufficiently provide the nutrients to develop autonomy, competence, and relatedness?

Extrinsic versus intrinsic motivation

One way in which SDT helps to develop our understanding of person-centred theory is in how it deals with how conditions of worth become internalized. Previously I used the term introjection as it is commonly used in person-centred theory. SDT makes the case, similar to Rogers (1959), that intrinsic motivation is necessarily autonomous, in the same way that a person with no conditions of worth would be free to be organismically guided. But this is not the case with extrinsic motivations. Ryan (1995) distinguished between four levels, beginning with external regulation where for example someone may do something out of fear of punishment. At the next level there is introjected regulation when the person may do something to avoid feeling guilty. Then there is identified regulation when the values of the action are endorsed), and finally integrated regulation where the person has integrated the identification with the self (see Table 4.4).

As such the term introjected is used in person-centred theory in the same way as integrated is used in SDT. SDT provides a more nuanced understanding of how conditions of worth can be viewed developmentally; beginning as externally regulated, as when a child does something to avoid punishment, becoming introjected, and finally identified and integrated. Through the process of therapy, as we shall see in the next chapter, this process is put into reverse.

Table 4.4 Levels of extrinsic regulation

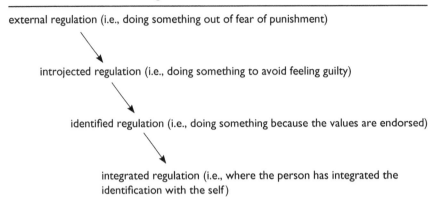

external regulation (i.e., doing something out of fear of punishment)

introjected regulation (i.e., doing something to avoid feeling guilty)

identified regulation (i.e., doing something because the values are endorsed)

integrated regulation (i.e., where the person has integrated the identification with the self)

Empirical evidence

First, one of the main findings in SDT research, replicated many times, and confirmed in meta-analysis, is that people are less likely to engage in activities that they find interesting when the rewards for that activity are extrinsic (e.g., money) (Deci, Koestner, & Ryan, 1999). But, when the social environment supports autonomy, for example through increased choice, then intrinsic motivation is enhanced (Reeve, Nix, & Hamm, 2003).

Second, Deci and Ryan (1995) distinguish between *true* or stable self-esteem and *contingent* or unstable self-esteem. A person is viewed as having true self-esteem when their attitudes, behaviours and feelings about themselves are self-determined (regulated by intrinsic motives), whereas they are considered to have contingent self-esteem when their attitudes, actions and feelings about themselves are dependent upon meeting external or introjected evaluative standards. Within this model, contingent self-evaluation is argued to be related to psychologically unhealthy, defensive and narcissistic traits. Thus, contingent self-evaluation seems to be similar to the Rogerian idea of self-regard being conditional upon introjected rules and values (Rogers, 1959), where the individual is seen to be guided more by external influences and introjected rules and values, in contrast to a more autonomous mode of functioning based on organismic valuing where the individual displays greater internal freedom regarding how they will act or respond.

Other research by Crocker and colleagues paints a similar picture, in which self-esteem is tied to certain domains of self-worth within which achievements or successful outcomes are perceived by the individual as essential to one's worth as a person (Crocker & Wolfe, 2001; Crocker, Luhtanen, Cooper, & Bouvrette, 2003). In other words, the external or integrated evaluative standards proposed by Deci and Ryan (1995) or the introjected rules and values (conditions of worth) proposed by Rogers (1959) are viewed as being linked to certain domains of life particularly valued or prized by the individual. The particular domains differ from person to person but include areas such as competition (the need to do better than others); specific competencies or abilities (e.g., academic); need for acceptance or approval from generalized others; need for family support; need for religious faith; and need to feel morally adequate or virtuous (Crocker & Wolfe, 2001; Crocker et al., 2003). Research with adolescents has shown evidence consistent with Rogers' view, with those adolescents experiencing greater conditional positive regard being less authentic and exhibiting more false-self behaviour (Harter, Marold, Whitesell, & Cobbs, 1996), and ill-being and resentment of parents (Assor, Roth, & Deci, 2004).

Third, research is supportive of the concept of the OVP. In a series of three studies, for example, Sheldon, Arndt, and Houser-Marko (2003) examined how people changed their mind over time about what goals and values to pursue. Their rationale was that evidence for the existence of an OVP would be demonstrated by people's tendency to move toward well-being related outcomes, such as those to do with intrinsic goals as opposed to extrinsic goals. Their results provide evidence that participants evidenced relatively greater ratings shifts towards goals that are more likely to be beneficial to their well-being.

Fourth, work into the longitudinal effects of self-concordant goal selection shows that those with more self-concordant goals (i.e., those who pursue goals for intrinsic rather than extrinsic reasons) put more sustained effort into those goals, which enables them to better attain those goals. Goal attainment in turn is associated with stronger feelings of autonomy, competence and relatedness, which in turn lead to greater well-being (Sheldon & Elliott, 1999). The evidence suggests that people grow when there is contact with the OVP. Other work shows that teenagers with mothers who are high in warmth and democratic parenting are more likely to hold intrinsic values and goals (Kasser, Ryan, Zax, & Sameroff, 1995; Williams, Cox, Hedberg, & Deci, 2000).

Finally, it is recognized that people have an intrinsic yearning to use their signature strengths (Seligman, 2004), and experience flow (Csikszentmihalyi, 1990; 1997). Although not explicitly stated, one can see how signature strengths could be seen as representative of the actualizing tendency: they are entirely consistent with who we are as individuals, we feel drawn to using our strengths, doing so intrinsically and for the fulfilment that they provide.

Such research as that briefly reviewed above is supportive of person-centred theory (for comprehensive reviews on the synergy between the person-centred approach and SDT, see Patterson & Joseph, 2007a; Sheldon, 2013). When we examine this weight of theory and evidence we see a real rapprochement between positive psychology and the person-centred approach, and the idea that the organismic valuing process needs to be set centre stage in a theory of helping. As Sheldon and Elliot (1999) wrote:

> . . . along with Rogers (1961), we believe that individuals have innate developmental trends and propensities that may be given voice by an organismic valueing process occurring within them. The voice can be very difficult to hear, but the current research suggests that the ability to hear it is of crucial importance for the pursuit of happiness. (p. 495)

Conclusion

As many positive psychologists ask about the application of SDT to therapy, it is clear that the theoretical groundwork is already well laid with over 50 years of theory and research on person-centred therapy. What positive psychology research tells us about personality processes is consistent with the person-centred approaches to therapy. The critical point here is that the locus of responsibility for the direction of the therapy is with the client, rather than with the therapist. It is self-evident that if the task of therapy is to help people to hear their own inner voice more clearly, then it is important that the voice of the therapist does not drown out the voice of the client. This is not to say that the therapist is silent, on the contrary, the therapist should be an active agent in the process of facilitating the client to listen to him or herself better. I shall go on to describe this in more detail in the next chapter. For the moment, however, what I want to emphasize is how revolutionary the implications of the person-centred approach are. The world is full of individuals and organizations that purport to know better than we do ourselves about how we should choose to live our lives, and what we should believe. The person-centred approach rejects this, and says instead that each of us is our own best expert on ourselves. In terms of therapeutic practice, it is the therapist's trust in the person's actualizing tendency which makes the person-centred approach so radically different from other therapeutic approaches. But psychologists who have not appreciated the profound significance of this view, that it is the client and not the therapist who knows best what direction to go in, often misunderstand client-centred psychotherapy. A common criticism of the client-centred approach is that if people knew best what direction to go in, then they would not need to seek help from a therapist. But this is to misunderstand the nature of the actualizing tendency as described by Rogers and the delicate artistry of the therapeutic approach itself. It is not easy to hear one's inner voice of wisdom, but the task is to help our clients to do just this. Positive psychologists, as we have seen, are re-examining the concept of the actualizing tendency, and the available evidence is consistent with the existence of an organismic valuing process that reliably guides us towards knowing our own best directions in life, and the steps that we should take to achieve our own optimal health and well-being.

Note

1 Self-actualization in person-centred theory refers to the development process and is not to be confused with Maslow's use of the same term to mean reaching a high level of functioning.

Further reading

Rogers, C. R. (1959). A theory of therapy, personality and interpersonal relationships, as developed in the client-centered framework. In S. Koch (Ed.), *Psychology: A study of a science, Vol. 3: Formulations of the person and the social context* (pp. 184–256). New York: McGraw Hill.

The most comprehensive of all Rogers' theoretical writings. Despite its date it remains the foundation of the person-centred approach.

Ryan, R. M., & Deci, E. L. (2000). Self-determination theory and the facilitation of intrinsic motivation, social development, and well-being. *American Psychologist, 55,* 68–78.

An overview and summary by the originators of self-determination theory.

Patterson, T. G., & Joseph, S. (2007a). Person-centered personality theory: Support from self-determination theory and positive psychology. *Journal of Humanistic Psychology, 47,* 117–139.

The paper that first summarized the research in SDT and how it supports the person-centred approach.

Cooper, M., & Joseph, S. (in press). Psychological foundations for humanistic psychotherapeutic practice. In D. A. Cain, K. Keenan, & S. Rubin (Eds), *Handbook of humanistic psychotherapies*. Washington, DC: American Psychiatric Association.

A comprehensive and up-to-date review of evidence in the psychological literature that has been overlooked but which supports humanistic therapies.

Chapter 5

The therapeutic relationship

In Chapter 4 I examined person-centred personality theory and some of the supporting evidence from positive psychology, concluding that person-centred theory provides us with a framework for understanding well-being. Person-centred theory, in turn, underlies the practice of person-centred therapy. Rogers' view was that given the right social-environmental conditions, clients' organismic valuing will be facilitated, thus they will be able to find their own directions, and that these directions will always be constructive, and towards becoming more fully functioning. Thus, what the therapist tries to do is to provide the right social-environmental conditions. In his highly regarded 1957 paper in the *Journal of Consulting Psychology*, Rogers described six conditions that he held were necessary and sufficient for positive therapeutic change. To this day it remains one of the most known of all of Rogers' writings. This chapter will provide an overview of the six conditions.

Six necessary and sufficient conditions

Rogers (1957) stated that there were six necessary and sufficient conditions, which, when present, provided the social environment that facilitated the OVP (see Table 5.1).

I. Contact between client and therapist

Condition 1 is referring to a precondition that, if not met, would mean that the following five conditions were redundant. What Rogers means by psychological contact is whether or not the two people are aware of each other, and that the behaviour of one impacts on the other. So, for example, with someone who is in a catatonic state, it would be difficult to judge whether there was psychological contact. For the relationship there has to be some degree of exchange between the parties in such a way that they impact on each other.

2. The client's incongruence

In the second condition, incongruence is explained as consisting of an incompatibility between underlying feelings and awareness of those feelings, or an incompatibility between awareness of feelings and the expression of feelings.

Table 5.1 The necessary and sufficient conditions of constructive personality change

1 Two persons are in psychological contact.
2 The first, whom we shall call the client, is in a state of incongruence, being vulnerable or anxious.
3 The second person, whom we shall call the therapist, is congruent or integrated in the relationship.
4 The therapist experiences unconditional positive regard for the client.
5 The therapist experiences an empathic understanding of the client's internal frame of reference and endeavours to communicate this experience to the client.
6 The communication to the client of the therapist's empathic understanding and unconditional positive regard is to a minimal degree achieved.

Source: Rogers, 1957, p. 96.

For example, someone who appears anxious to an observer but has no awareness themselves of feeling anxious would be said to be incongruent in terms of their underlying feelings and their awareness of those feelings. Someone who is aware of their anxiety but says that they are feeling relaxed would be said to be incongruent between awareness and expression.

3. The therapist's congruence

In the third condition, the therapist is congruent, that is to say, he or she is aware of their inner experience, e.g., feelings of anger or sadness, and is able to express this openly and honestly if thought to be appropriate. This refers to the authenticity of the therapist, that is to say their ability to know themselves and to be able to be genuine.

4. The therapist's unconditional positive regard

In the fourth condition, the therapist is able to provide unconditional positive regard, that is to say, he or she is able to accept the client without imposing conditions of worth on the client. This is the theoretical crux of the therapy, and as we discussed in the previous chapters relates to the idea of respecting the client's right to self-determination.

5. The therapist's empathic understanding

In the fifth condition, the therapist has empathic understanding: that is to say, he or she is able to sense what the client's experience is like. This refers to the therapist's ability to show the client that he or she is with them, attempting to understand their point of view.

6. The client's perception of the conditions

Finally, in the sixth condition, the client perceives the therapist's empathy and unconditional acceptance. This is the notion that while the therapist must endeavour to be congruent, empathic and unconditionally accepting, ultimately it is the client who must experience the therapist as congruent, and themselves as understood and unconditionally valued if the therapy is to make a difference for them.

An attitude not a technique

Rogers believed that if these six conditions described above were in existence then constructive personality change would occur, but only if all six were present, and the more that they were present the more marked would be the constructive personality change of the client.

The six necessary and sufficient conditions outlined by Rogers (1957) describe the attitudinal qualities of the person-centred psychotherapist, their congruence, empathy, and unconditional positive regard. Conditions 3, 4, and 5 are sometimes referred to as the *core conditions*. These describe the attitude of the person-centred therapist – they endeavour to be congruent, empathic, and to experience unconditional positive regard for their client. Empathy is central to practice because the best vantage point for understanding behaviour is from the internal frame of reference of the individual themselves. Rogers (1951) argued that the only way we could understand another person's behaviour was to see the world through their eyes. Then, even the most seemingly bizarre behaviour would make meaningful sense.

Robbins (2015), a contemporary humanistic psychologist, describes how these core conditions operate as a unified force for healing that is, as he says, the perfect example of the application of the neo-Aristotelian concept of virtue.

> Rogers (1961) found that the virtuous therapist is one who cultivates a growth-promoting climate through the acquisition of three essential traits: congruency, unconditional positive regard for the client and empathic understanding. Notice that these virtues are interdependent. For example, empathic understanding can be used by psychopaths as a means to manipulate and control other people, but when coupled with unconditional positive regard, empathy becomes a benevolent and powerful conduit for interpersonal healing. A congruent therapist may have the integrity and honesty to confront a client about his or her faults, but without unconditional positive regard and empathy, these confrontations are likely to be harsh and damaging rather than constructive avenues for therapeutic change. Although Rogers did not explicitly recognize his approach to therapy as grounded in a neo-Aristotelian conception of virtue, his work nevertheless provides a perfect example of its application. (Robbins, 2015, p. 40)

Rogers wrote his 1957 paper as an integrative statement about therapeutic personality change in any successful therapy. As such, Rogers was saying that all psychotherapies are effective insofar as the necessary and sufficient conditions are present. The 1957 paper of Rogers remains a cornerstone of person-centred theory and practice (see, e.g., Bozarth & Wilkins, 2001; Haugh & Merry, 2001; Wyatt, 2001; Wyatt & Sanders, 2001). Most psychologists regardless of their therapeutic approach agree that these conditions are important, and that the therapeutic relationship needs to be developed. However, this might be for different reasons.

Broadly speaking there are three main reasons (Murphy & Joseph, 2013). First is the view that the therapeutic relationship creates rapport between the client and therapist in order to increase compliance on the part of the client with the treatment provided. This view considers the therapeutic relationship to be important but not directly causal in therapeutic outcome, and is the approach commonly employed by therapists offering cognitive-behavioural techniques. Second is the psychoanalytically derived view that the therapeutic relationship is important because it is the vehicle for the delivery of the treatment and as such does contribute to outcome because it enables unconscious processes in the client to be made conscious. The relationship between client and therapist is constructed in order to create a particular environmental climate in which the client is often frustrated into projecting their unresolved unconscious parts of their experiences onto the therapist. Third is the person-centred view that the therapeutic relationship is directly causal in therapeutic change because the relationship is considered to *be* the therapy. Here the therapist's task in the relationship is to communicate understanding and acceptance.

Contemporary perspectives

The language of Rogers' conditions can, for some, seem outdated and fail to convey a vivid picture of what the experience of being in such a relationship is like – the sense of connectedness and immersion that results. As such, finding new ways to talk about the core conditions can be useful. One concept which has helped us understand the power of the conditions is that of *relational depth*.

Relational depth

Relational depth is defined as:

> A state of profound contact and engagement between two people, in which each person is fully real with the Other, and able to understand and value the Other's experience at a high level. (Mearns & Cooper, 2005, p. xii)

Relational depth is what unfolds when a therapist offers the conditions to a high degree. As such it does not necessarily describe anything new but allows us to understand empathy, congruence and unconditional positive regard and the depth of relationship that results when these conditions are experienced together in full force (Mearns, 2013; Sanders, 2013).

Emotional Intelligence

It is also helpful to think of person-centred therapy as a profound experiential approach founded on the emotional intelligence of the therapist. The basis of the person-centred therapeutic approach is Condition 3, the therapist's congruence. Congruence refers to the person's awareness of their underlying thoughts and feelings, and their ability to express these thoughts and feelings appropriately in the context (Bozarth, 1998; Wyatt, 2001). That is to say, there is congruence between the internal cognitive and emotional states of the person, their conscious awareness of those states, and their ability to articulate the expression of those states.

Congruence, when combined with Condition 5, empathic understanding, would involve all four facets of emotional intelligence as discussed by Salovey, Caruso, & Mayer, 2004; Salovey, Mayer, & Caruso, 2002). The congruent therapist who has an empathic understanding of the client's frame of reference is: (1) perceptive of how the client is feeling; (2) of how they themselves are feeling; (3) able to manage their own emotions and to use their own emotions creatively in the service of the therapeutic relationship; and (4) they are able to understand emotions and to label them appropriately.

Authentic relationship

What I want to emphasize most of all is how person-centred therapy allows for tremendous variety and spontaneity in ways of working. No two person-centred therapists will be the same, as it is an approach to therapy that is founded on the therapists' emotional intelligence. Essentially, the idea is that within an authentic, accepting and emotionally literate relationship, people are able to drop their defences and get to know themselves better, and feel free to make new choices in life. Person-centred theory says that, in such relationships, people move to make new and wiser choices for themselves by listening more to their organismic valuing process, the inner voice of wisdom within us all. What this means in practice is that the person-centred therapist is someone who has a deep understanding of themselves and is able to be present in an authentic way with the client. The therapist strives to understand the client's world from the client's perspective, and they are accepting of the client's directions in life without imposing their own agenda, that is to say, the self-determination of the client is paramount.

Self-determination

This latter point, being accepting of the client's directions without imposing one's own, is as we have seen already, the crux of client-centred therapy (i.e. Condition 4) and is communicated through the therapist's congruence and empathy (see Bozarth, 1998). It is fundamental to the client-centred therapist, because of his or her trust in the actualizing tendency as the one central source of human motivation, that they do not intervene, and have no intention of intervening. As Bozarth (1998) said:

> The therapist goes with the client, goes at the client's pace, goes with the client in his/her own ways of thinking, of experiencing, or processing. The therapist cannot be up to other things, have other intentions without violating the essence of person-centred therapy. To be up to other things – whatever they might be – is a 'yes, but' reaction to the essence of the approach. It must mean that when the therapist has intentions of treatment plans, of treatment goals, of interventive strategies to get the client somewhere or for the client to do a certain thing, the therapist violates the essence of person-centred therapy. (pp. 11–12)

Education of therapists

A final topic for this section is how the person-centred approach offers a different view of the education of therapists. As person-centred therapists we bring ourselves into the therapeutic relationship. Rather than the emphasis on training in techniques for specific problems there is a need for greater attention to therapist's personal development, their ability to accept others, and to be alongside another person and to understand the world through their eyes. As we have seen, most of the success in therapy comes through the client's own resources, and their relationship with the therapist. As such, it is the qualities of the therapist, their empathy and their congruence that should be the focus of their education, not so much the techniques they use.

Process of therapeutic change

For change to occur within the client the combination of the conditions is important as described above, but each condition plays a particular role. As we have seen in the previous chapter, person-centred theory says that problems in living arise through conditions of worth. So it is that the six necessary and sufficient conditions are therapeutic because they offer an unconditionally accepting environment. But it is no use the therapist only having an unconditionally accepting attitude, unless the client experiences it as such. This is where the therapist's empathy and congruence come in, since these are the vehicles for the transmission of unconditional positive regard.

In his 1959 paper, Rogers described the process through which the conditions are healing. The process is summarized as follows:

1   In order for the process of 'defense' to be reversed – for a customarily 'threatening experience' to be 'accurately symbolized' in 'awareness' and assimilated into the 'self-structure', certain conditions must exist.

     a   There must be a decrease in the 'conditions of worth'.
     b   There must be an increase in unconditional 'self-regard'.

2   The communicated 'unconditional positive regard' of a significant other is one way of achieving these conditions.

     a   In order for the 'unconditional positive regard' of a significant other to be communicated, it must exist in a context of 'empathic' understanding.
     b   When the individual 'perceives' such 'unconditional positive regard', existing 'conditions of worth' are weakened or dissolved.
     c   Another consequence is the increase in his own 'unconditional positive self-regard'.
     d   Conditions 2a and 2b above thus being met, 'threat' is reduced, the process of 'defense is reversed', and 'experiences' customarily 'threatening' are 'accurately symbolized' and integrated into the self concept. (p. 230)

The crux of person-centred therapy, therefore, is the provision, by the therapist, to the client, of an unconditionally accepting social environment. As we have seen in the previous chapter, psychological problems arise as a result of the internalization of conditions of worth. The person-centred therapist, in offering the core conditions to their client, is able to offer a social environment that serves to dissolve the client's conditions of worth. As the client begins to feel unconditionally accepted in the therapeutic relationship, perhaps for the first time in his or her life, he or she is able to begin to develop unconditional self-acceptance. As Bozarth wrote:

> The individual's return to unconditional positive self-regard is the crux of psychological growth in the theory. It is the factor that reunifies the self with the actualizing tendency . . . Rogers hypothesises that one must perceive reception of unconditional positive regard in order to correct the pathological state. The communication of unconditional positive regard by a significant other is one way to achieve the above conditions. (1998, p. 84)

Perceiving oneself as unconditionally accepted, not feeling that there are conditions of worth to live up to, opens up the possibility for people to begin to evaluate experiences organismically. The notion of the OVP is illustrated by Maslow who described how he would encourage his students to learn for themselves to listen to their own voices:

> I sometimes suggest to my students that when they are given a glass of wine and asked how they like it, they try a different way of responding. First, I suggest that they not look at the label on the bottle. Thus they will *not* use it to get any cue about whether or not they *should* like it. Next, I recommend that they close their eyes if possible and that they 'make a hush'. Now they are ready to look within themselves and try to shut out the noise of the world so that they may savor the wine on their tongues and look to the 'Supreme Court' inside themselves. (1993, pp. 44–45)

The point is to learn to let the direction of our lives be guided by the 'Supreme Court' inside ourselves. As we have seen, the OVP is an idea founded on the assumption that when people listen to their inner wisdom, constructive behaviour and not destructive behaviour is the result, because in essence people are motivated by the tendency towards actualization. When people lead lives directed by their inner wisdom, they are, these humanistic theories say, self-directed, creative, autonomous, social, have an accurate view of themselves and other people, are willing to try and understand other people's points of view, and are open to new experiences. In Maslow's terminology, such people move towards self-actualization:

> They listen to their own voices; they take responsibility; they are honest; and they work hard. They find out who they are and what they are, not only in terms of their mission in life, but also in terms of the way their feet hurt when they wear such and such a pair of shoes and whether they do or do not like eggplant. . . . All this is what the real self means. (1993, p. 49)

Table 5.2 Theoretical process of client-centred therapy

Conditions of worth
⇓
Denial and distortion of experience
⇓
Inauthenticity
⇓
Client-centred psychotherapy
⇓
Dissolves conditions of worth
⇓
Unconditional positive self-regard
⇓
Experiences no longer distorted and denied
⇓
Greater authenticity
⇓
Movement towards becoming fully functioning

In Rogers' terms, they move towards fully functioning. So the essence of therapy is helping people to be in contact with their OVP by countering the many forces acting on them that prevent them from being guided by their OVP – notably conditional regard. In sum, the heart of person-centred therapy is the ability of the therapist to experience unconditional positive regard for the client. The process of therapy is shown in Table 5.2.

Unconditional positive regard must surely be one of the most misunderstood concepts in psychotherapy and counselling. As Rogers (1957) wrote:

> It is probably evident from the description that completely unconditional positive regard would never exist except in theory. From a clinical and experiential point of view I believe that the most accurate statement is that the effective therapist experiences unconditional positive regard for the client during many moments of his contact with him, yet from time to time he experiences only a conditional positive regard – and perhaps at times a negative regard, though this is not likely in effective therapy. It is in this sense that unconditional positive regard exists as a matter of degree in any relationship. (Rogers, 1957, cited in Kirchenbaum, 2007, p. 225)

It is true that practically all therapists say that they value and use these person-centred conditions. But it is the belief in the actualizing tendency that provides the theoretical rationale for the therapeutic provision of an unconditionally accepting attitude, empathy and congruence.

> It is the belief in the actualising tendency that sets client-centred psychotherapy apart from other therapy traditions. It might be said that the actualising tendency

is to client-centred psychotherapy what the unconscious is to psychoanalysis. It would be nonsense for a therapist to claim to practise psychoanalysis just because they used free association techniques if they did not also believe that there were unconscious forces shaping behaviour. Similarly, it would be nonsense for therapists to claim to practise client-centred psychotherapy just because they endeavour to accept their client unconditionally if they do not hold in the first place that there is an actualising tendency. (Joseph, 2003a, p. 305)

Thus, in my view, the crux of person-centred therapy is not the therapist's attitudinal conditions per se that characterize person-centred therapy, but holding these attitudes in conjunction with the meta-theoretical assumption that people are intrinsically motivated towards constructive and optimal functioning and that under the right social-environmental conditions this force is released. As Grant wrote:

Client-centered therapists make no assumptions about what people need or how they should be free. They do not attempt to promote self-acceptance, self-direction, positive growth, self-actualization, congruence between real or perceived selves, a particular vision of reality, or anything. . . . *Client-centered therapy is the practice of simply respecting the right to self-determination of others.* (2004, p.158)

It is that respect for the self-determination of others that underpins the unconditional attitude of the therapist and the principled stance of non-directivity, which is the distinguishing feature of the approach (see, Levitt, 2005a). As Brodley (2005a) wrote:

The non-directive attitude is psychologically profound; it is not a technique. Early in a therapist's development it may be superficial and prescriptive – 'Don't do this' or 'Don't do that'. But with time, self-examination and therapy experience, it becomes an aspect of the therapist's character. It represents a feeling of profound respect for the constructive potential in persons and great sensitivity to their vulnerability. (p. 3)

In summary, these core attitudinal qualities of the therapist only make sense in relation to the meta-theoretical perspective of person-centred theory. Endeavouring to be empathic, congruent and unconditionally accepting is not in itself client-centred therapy: one must also hold and respect that the actualizing tendency is the client's source of motivation. Belief in the actualizing tendency has profound implications for practice. A therapist endeavouring to hold the conditions of empathy, congruence and unconditional positive regard, but who is not trusting in this one central source of energy in the human organism – the actualizing tendency – is not practising person-centred therapy. It is the client-centred psychotherapist's trust in the actualizing tendency that makes the approach so revolutionary (Bozarth, 1998).

Imagine what it is like to be in such a relationship as described by Rogers' six conditions, in which you perceive yourself to be accepted, valued and understood. The therapist Robert Wicks tells a story of how at the end of a series of sessions with a client he was asking her some final questions to wrap up their time together. He hoped that the questions would help her frame the learning that she had got through therapy. Her response about the changes she had made was positive, so Wicks asked her what had helped her get to this new point in her life:

> 'Well,' she said, 'it was simple.'
>
> 'Simple?' I replied. . . .
>
> 'Yes. You see, the first time I came in here to see you, I simply watched how you sat with me; then I began sitting with myself in the same way.' (Wicks, 2008, p. 4)

In reflecting on this experience with this client, Wicks asks what it is that people experience when they are with therapists.

> Do they experience a sense of respectful space where they can rest their burdens, anger, questions, projections, stress, anxiety, and wonder? Or, do they feel our sense of exhaustion, need to always be right or in control, or even our desire to be viewed as wise, attractive, witty, or helpful? What do people feel when they are with us? (2008, p. 5)

Although it is not often made explicit, person-centred therapies have much in common with therapeutic approaches derived from Eastern traditions. The relation between the person-centred approach and the tradition of Zen is explored elsewhere by Brazier (1995) who discusses how Zen is a form of therapy:

> The challenge which Zen poses us is to reach deeply into the experience of being alive to find something authentic. . . . Zen is simply the awakening of one heart by another, of sincerity by sincerity. Although words can express it, and can point to it, they cannot substitute for it. It is the authentic experience which occurs when concern with all that is inessential drops away. (pp. 12–13)

This sounds consistent with person-centred therapy. It too might be said to be the awakening of one heart by another, of the experience of being empathetically understood, unconditionally accepted and genuinely received. The point I am making is that person-centred therapy is not a technical form of therapy in which there are techniques employed and manualized steps to follow, but an approach to therapy which is deeply relational as described by the six necessary and sufficient conditions.

In the same vein, I would also say that person-centred therapy with its stance of going with the client has the potential to be a deeply existential approach. A similar argument was made by Bretherton and Ørner (2003) who said:

the most obvious way in which the existential approach parallels positive psychotherapy is in its preoccupation with what is presented by the client rather than with global models of deficit and disorder. Using the phenomenological method, therapists attempt to 'bracket' (put to one side) many of the assumptions and reactions they have with regard to clients (including the desire for therapeutic progress) so as to better engage with a client's way of being. By stepping back from their own prejudices and stereotypes, existential therapists can identify client's possibilities as well as their limitations . . . The existentialists suggest that by identifying the constellations of meaning by which we relate to the world, we give ourselves the opportunity of decision – to decide whether to alter our way of being in the world. (p. 136; see also Bretherton & Ørner, 2004)

Similarly, Deurzen (1998) said:

Radical existential psychotherapy focuses on the inter-personal and supra-personal dimensions, as it tries to capture and question people's worldviews. Such existential work aims at clarifying and understanding personal values and beliefs, making explicit what was previously implicit and unsaid. Its practice is primarily philosophical and seeks to enable a person to live more deliberately, more authentically and more purposefully, whilst accepting the limitations and contradictions of human existence . . . Existential psychotherapy has to be reinvented and recreated by every therapist and with every new client. It is essentially about investigating human existence and the particular preoccupations of one individual and this has to be done without preconceptions or set ways of proceeding. There has to be complete openness to the individual situation and an attitude of wonder that will allow the specific circumstances and experiences to unfold in their own right. (pp. 13–14).

Does person-centred therapy work?

A central question is whether or not person-centred psychotherapy is an effective way of helping people. Early research throughout the 1960s provided evidence consistent with Rogers' hypothesis of the necessary and sufficient conditions (Truax & Mitchell, 1971; see Barrett-Lennard, 1998). However, over the next two decades the research tradition in person-centred psychotherapy dwindled, in large part because the new generation of research active psychologists tended to be interested in the new cognitive approach to psychotherapy, and person-centred psychotherapy became increasingly a marginalized approach within mainstream psychology (for the reasons already described in Chapter 4, see also Bohart, O'Hara, & Leitner, 1998). Even so, a substantial body of research has in fact developed over the past 50 years which testifies to the effectiveness of person-centred therapy.

Recently, the evidence for person-centred therapy was reviewed by Murphy and Joseph (in press). First, they summarized the literature spanning 1940 to 2000. The very early research of the 1940s concerned the role of non-directivity and how it facilitated self-exploration. As the theory developed into the 1950s and onwards, research began to investigate the six necessary and sufficient conditions. Smith, Glass, and Miller (1980) conducted the first meta-analysis of psychotherapy and this included a review of studies of person-centred therapy, concluding with their now famous dodo bird verdict, that the well established main therapies were equivalent. A later meta-analysis of outcome studies was carried out by Greenberg, Elliott, and Lietaer (1994) reaching the same conclusion and was equally supportive of person-centred therapy.

However, as Murphy and Joseph (in press) note, the 1980s and 1990s were a time when research in the person-centred approach had dwindled from its initial peak in the 1950s. A new question was being asked which was how therapies performed in relation to medical model diagnostic categories. Such research required massive expenditure to fund randomized controlled studies, but as the person-centred approach was now only marginally represented in universities and institutions where such research was conducted it struggled to compete.

Reviewing the literature post 2000, Murphy and Joseph (in press) note the evidence for the effectiveness of person-centred therapy has, however, continued to build. More recent studies have begun to address the knowledge gap in relation to practice-based evidence (Stiles, Barkham, Twigg, Mellor-Clark, & Cooper, 2006) and diagnostically defined outcomes and evidence from meta-analytic studies continue to support the dodo bird verdict (Elliott, Greenberg, Watson, Timulak, & Freire, 2013).

There is no doubt that therapy works, but how does it work? Decades of therapy research suggest that Rogers (1957) statement was close to the mark in pointing to the central importance of the therapeutic relationship (see Martin, Garske, & Davis, 2000; Wampold, 2001). It is known that successful therapy is not due to particular therapeutic techniques, levels of training, or the use of diagnosis. Over a decade ago the American Psychological Association Division 29 Task Force on empirically Supported Therapy Relationships (Norcross, 2001) concluded that it is the therapeutic relationship and the client's own inner resources that are important. This is a conclusion now reached by many researchers (e.g. Bozarth, 1998; Bozarth & Motomasa, 2005; Cornelius-White, 2002; Duncan & Miller, 2000; Hubble & Miller, 2004; Martin et al., 2000; Wampold, 2001). Clients themselves often report on the importance to them of a trusting, safe and non judgemental therapeutic relationship (Chouliara et al., 2012).

Further, analyses of the factors that contribute to the development of a positive working alliance (i.e. effective therapeutic relationship) also accord with the central tenets of client-centred therapy. For example, therapists' personal qualities of being flexible, honest, respectful, trustworthy, confident, warm, interested and open have been shown to contribute positively to a better working alliance. Therapist techniques of exploration, reflection, noting past therapy success, accurate interpretation, facilitating expression of affect and attending to the client's experience also contribute positively to the alliance (see Ackerman & Hilsenroth, 2003).

In recent years there has been interest in self-compassion, with evidence that individuals who are more self-compassionate having healthier and more productive lives than those who are self-critical (Neff, 2003; Neff & Vonk, 2009; Gilbert & Irons, 2009). As a psychological construct, self-compassion is defined as being able to treat oneself with kindness and involves accepting painful thoughts and feelings without being judgemental or self-pitying (Neff, Kirkpatrick, & Rude, 2007). There is a clear conceptual similarity between self-compassion and unconditional positive self-regard as both reflecting healthier ways of relating to oneself.

As we have seen, person-centred therapy is first and foremost about the relationship and how the inner resources of the client can be brought to the fore. Research has pointed to the role of the client in successful therapeutic outcome, suggesting that as much as 40–87 per cent of outcome variance may be attributable to client factors alone, followed by relationship factors, with therapeutic orientation coming a distant third place (Bozarth & Motomasa, 2005; Duncan & Miller, 2000; Hubble & Miller, 2004; Wampold, 2001). Clearly, the client seems to have been unduly forgotten in psychotherapy research, and positive psychological approaches to therapy are helping to reintroduce a consideration of the impact of the client into scientific research protocols (Hubble & Miller, 2004).

With positive psychology we are also now entering a new era of research in which there is again interest in relationship factors. Various psychometric tools based on person-centred theory can be used to test aspects of personal centred theory. For example, one of the most widely used measures is the Barrett-Lennard Relationship Inventory (BLRI: Barett-Lennard, 1986). The BLRI can be used to assess perceptions of empathy, congruence and unconditional positive regard from the clients perspective, and how these perceptions relate to later outcome (see Table 5.3 for example items).

Other tools developed more recently include the Wilczynski, Brodley, and Brody (2008) rating system for studying non-directive client-centred interviews, and the Person-Centred and Experiential Psychotherapy Scale (PCEPS: Freire, Elliott, & Westwell, 2013). Raters can use these scales to assess the extent to which a therapist's responses are consistent with person-centred practice. Using such tools we can begin to investigate whether ratings on such scales relate to better outcomes.

In an example of small scale research into post-traumatic growth, one such study asked clients in group therapy for interpersonal trauma to complete the BLRI in order to test whether their scores were related to outcome (Payne,

Table 5.3 Example items from the BLRI

My therapist wants to understand how I see things.
My therapist nearly always knows exactly what I mean.
I feel that my therapist is real and genuine with me.
My therapist is friendly and warm with me.
I feel that my therapist really values me.
My therapist is openly himself/herself in our relationship.

Liebling-Kalifani, & Joseph, 2007). Consistent with the six conditions, it was hypothesized that those who scored higher on the BLRI would do better subsequently on various tools to assess their psychological functioning. Evidence was consistent with this. As a small pilot study this work provokes new ideas for research in which one assesses the degree to which clients experience the core conditions during therapy in order to test how these assessments relate to subsequent functioning.

Conclusion

In this chapter the statement by Rogers that there are six necessary and sufficient conditions for therapeutic change was examined, put into a contemporary context and discussed in relation to the theory of process and the evidence for effectiveness of therapy. In the person-centred approach, the therapeutic relationship matters as a way of transmitting unconditional acceptance. Person-centred and related therapies are based on the notion of going with the client's direction. As such it is often understood that the use of therapeutic techniques such as relaxation exercises is incompatible with the person-centred approach. My view is that it is not the use of techniques per se that is incompatible but the introduction by the therapist of anything that interferes with the self-determination of the client. Anything that supports the self-determination of the client and their direction in that moment is by definition person-centred. Seen this way it seems to me that there may be instances throughout therapy when experiences may be introduced by the therapist, but these cannot be determined in advance by the therapist. This will be the theme of the next chapter as I go on to develop the idea of positive therapy.

Further reading

Rogers, C. R. (1957). The necessary and sufficient conditions of therapeutic personality change. *Journal of Consulting Psychology, 21*, 95–103.
This is the paper that first set out the conditions for the therapeutic relationship and which for many remains the cornerstone of therapeutic practice.

Mearns, D., & Cooper, M. (2005). *Working at relational depth in counselling and psychotherapy*. London: Sage.
This is the book that introduced the concept of relational depth to the world. Whether relational depth offers a different view from that of Rogers remains a point for discussion, but it certainly brings the idea of the therapeutic relationship to life in a new way.

Murphy, D., & Joseph, S. (in press). Person-centered therapy: past, present and future orientation. In D. A. Cain, K. Keenan, & S. Ruban (Eds), *Handbook of humanistic psychotherapies*. Washington, DC: American Psychiatric Association.
A comprehensive review of the evidence for person-centred therapy. The evidence is good that it works.

Worsley, R., & Joseph, S. (2007), (Eds), *Person-centred practice: Case studies in positive psychology*. Ross-on-Wye: PCCS books.
If you are used to thinking of therapy as a set of techniques to be learned, this book will show you what person-centred practice looks like. A series of case studies by leading practitioners describing their therapeutic relationships with their clients.

Chapter 6

Process direction and person-activity fit

In the previous chapter, I discussed person-centred therapy and how it was a relationship-based approach derived from the notion of following the lead of the client rather than an intervention with specified techniques to deliver. Does this mean that techniques cannot be used? In my view techniques may be used but it is how one uses them that is important. As Yalom (2001) writes:

> the flow of therapy should be spontaneous, forever following unanticipated riverbeds: it is grotesquely distorted by being packaged into a formula . . . I try to avoid technique that is prefabricated and do best if I allow my choices to flow spontaneously. (pp. 34–35)

The person-centred therapist is non-directive in the sense that they do not want to interfere with the direction of the client. But non-directivity is a confusing concept because while it tells us what not to do it does not tell us what to do. A helpful way to consider the concept of non-directivity is to see it as only one side of a coin. The other side of that coin is the client's direction. The therapist is non-directive because he or she is following the client's direction. When Rogers decided to stop using the term non-directivity and replace it with the term person-centred this was the point he was making.

The term self-determination fulfils a similar purpose as the term client-centred in helping us to understand that positive therapy is about supporting the needs of the client. We have seen already that person-centred psychology is supported by self-determination theory and research providing us with a solid foundation for a positive psychology of psychotherapy.

Drawing on positive psychology research, there are a tremendous amount of techniques that clients might sometimes find useful (see, e.g., Joseph, 2015; Lopez & Snyder, 2009). Although the use of techniques has been a contentious issue among person-centred therapists because of the confusion around the concept of non-directivity, the issue is not whether techniques may be used, but how they are used. The positive therapist should be free to draw on the wider resources available to them, as long as they are able to articulate how the use of particular tests or techniques respects the self-determination of the client and helps to facilitate contact with their OVP. As Yalom says in the quote above it is about spontaneous flow and working in a way that is not wedded to the use of any one particular set of techniques, but rather coming from an attitudinal base characterized by the conditions described in the previous chapter.

Seligman (2002) and Seligman and Peterson (2003) originally discussed what they see as positive therapy and positive clinical psychology. Their central contention is that much of what makes therapy successful is what they refer to as the 'deep strategies', such as instilling hope, providing narration and building strengths (such as courage, rationality and capacity for pleasure). It is implicit in the person-centred approach to positive therapy that the deep strategies can come from the client themselves as contact with their OVP develops.

In this sense, positive therapy, as I am defining it, is person-centred because of its theoretical base in the notion of the actualizing tendency, and thus the unconditional therapeutic relationship as a means to support the client's developmental process of becoming, but at the same time and without contravening the unconditionality of the relationship, the therapist is open to the possibility of introducing experiences into the therapy session that can support the autonomy, relatedness and competence of the client.

As such positive therapy requires a great ability to listen – really listen – and the artistry to go with the flow of the client and for the therapist to bring themselves, their knowledge and skills to the service of the client. Many therapists will recognize the similarity with this view and that of the notion of process direction.

Using process direction

Worsley (2009) is the major exponent of the more process-oriented approach to person-centred therapy. When thinking about what happens in therapy, he likens the client's process to the 'how' as opposed to the content of what the client says, the 'what'. His view is that is it equally person-centred to address both the how and the what. As such, sometimes the therapist's intuition may lead. As Worsley writes:

> The image that occurs to me is of two people in a dark tunnel, each equipped with a flashlight. From time to time, the therapist is able to shine the beam further ahead than the client. (On many more occasions it is the client who can do this. In any case, what is actually seen in the pool of light is always for the client to determine.). . . . He may step out ahead, but then must await the client's judgement upon what he has done. (2009, p. 31)

Worsley argues that it is possible to use theory from other branches of humanistic psychology without the therapy becoming directive. He gives the example of using ideas from Transactional Analysis (TA), with a client who was already using this language of his own accord. Similarly, from my own experience I gave the example of Teresa. Teresa had gone to see a therapist because she often had problems with her line manager at work which was causing her anxiety. Her line manager is a middle-aged man and Teresa is a young women in her twenties. Teresa experiences her line manager as very controlling. In meetings, she often finds herself becoming confused and feeling patronised. She feels angry but tries to hide her anger, becoming tearful, often causing problems among her team workers who cannot understand Teresa's reactions. During one session, Teresa mentioned to her therapist that when she was a student she had read the book by Eric Berne, *Games People Play*, which one of her flatmates had had. This opened up conversation and the therapist offered to say a bit more about the ideas of Eric Berne, which Teresa welcomed. At this point it was helpful that the therapist had a knowledge of TA and could introduce it into the session.

The example of TA

Eric Berne introduced a system of therapy known as Transactional Analysis (TA). This is a complex theoretical system, a portion of which is what is called the ego state model. This consists of three ego states: the child, the parent and the adult. In our child ego state, we think and feel in a way like we did when we were children. In our parent ego state, we think and feel in a way like those of the significant parental figures from our childhood. In our adult ego state, we think and feel in ways that are direct responses to the here and now environment.

Parental states can be nurturing or controlling, and child states can be free or adapted. The nurturing parent corresponds to those aspects of parenting activity that have promoted growth and fostered autonomy. The controlling parent is the voice that criticizes behaviour. Any behaviour is driven by the ego state that is in control of the personality at that moment. Normally, Berne argued, we move in and out of these different ego states. We can analyse interpersonal interactions in terms of the communication between individuals at an ego state level of analysis. Often, at a social level, it might appear that we are talking adult to adult, but at the psychological level, something else is happening. For example, we are talking parent to child, or child to parent. In TA there is the recognition that messages from one person to another can operate on two levels, which Berne referred to as the social level and the psychological level. The social level refers to what we say to one another whereas the psychological level refers to what we really mean. When the social and the psychological levels are incongruent in this way, the psychological message is said to be *ulterior*. Berne maintained that the psychological message was always the real message, and it was at this psychological level that the course of events was always determined. People would act in ways that were guided by their real values, motives and intentions, not by those values, motives and intentions that they pretended to hold (see Stewart, 1989).

By talking to Teresa about the language of ego states, the therapist was able to help her explore her issues from this new perspective. Through the TA framework, Teresa began to understand how her line manager spoke to her at the social level as adult to adult, but further exploration showed how at the ulterior level he would be communicating from parent to her child, leaving Teresa confused and bewildered. As Teresa began to realize this, she felt empowered in her interactions and began to explore new ways of remaining in the adult ego state when her line manager invited her into the child ego state.

The therapist in this case was not a specialist in TA but was able to go with Teresa's direction as the topic was introduced by her and, as Worsley says in the quote above, shine a beam of light ahead which Teresa was able to make use of. TA offers techniques and ways of thinking that can be useful to clients in thinking about how their problems in living arose and are maintained in everyday life.

Above I have described positive therapy as a broad meta-theoretical approach that is person-centred in its philosophy of always going with the client's direction and supporting their needs for self-determination through the use of the relationship conditions. As such it is not a prescribed approach but one that allows for spontaneous flow. In the above example, ideas from TA were used. In this way, the positive therapist is able to introduce experiences into the therapy session. If the therapist is truly able to go with the flow of the client then they need to be responsive to whatever it is the client is bringing.

The point is that the positive therapist should be able to follow the unanticipated riverbeds. Knowledge of different therapeutic approaches is valuable, as will be an engagement with contemporary positive psychology techniques. Recent scholarship in positive psychology also points to the same conclusion – that no one technique is suitable all of the time for all people, but that we need to assess person-activity fit.

Person-activity fit and positive psychology techniques

One observation from positive psychology is the recognition that not all interventions will suit everyone (Lyubomirsky, 2008). Person-centred theory helps us to develop this notion further by saying that it will be the client who will know best for themselves what they need. So rather than the therapist trying to fit the client into one of several pre-specified options for exercises, the therapist follows the client's lead and co-creates something unique for that person.

As such, positive therapy as I envisage it is a philosophical relational stance rather than the collection of a specific set of exercises or techniques to be applied. It is a philosophical stance based on Rogers' (1957) paper on the six necessary and sufficient conditions of personality change in which the therapist endeavours to be empathic, congruent and unconditionally regarding. That is what the therapist strives to achieve, nothing more. This can be hard for some people to understand as they are used to thinking of therapy as a set of techniques or exercises. What it means, however, is that the repertoire of the therapist is not restricted to any one set of techniques but open to the range of techniques and exercises that are available.

But this is not the same as eclecticism as the therapist is always working in a way consistent with non-directive person-centred therapy. Reconciling the notion of using exercises and techniques with the notion of non-directivity, Grant (1990) suggests that from a principled position of non-directivity the therapist should be prepared to do whatever it takes in service to the client based on their need at that moment in therapy. In short, insofar as the therapist is using exercises and techniques in such a way that they are maintaining their unconditional acceptance and respect for the client's self-determination, it is possible to use techniques and exercises.

I hope to have illustrated in this discussion how although person-centred practitioners are often set against the use of exercises and techniques when they are used to direct the client, there is nothing inconsistent with introducing experiences for the client within the person-centred framework. What is important is the therapist's underlying philosophical stance. It is not what the therapist does that is important, it is *how* they do it.

Positive psychology experiences

Positive psychology has built up an impressive body of knowledge concerning various factors such as curiosity, gratitude, forgiveness, and so on, showing how they are generally adaptive mechanisms for a happier life. Based on the research a variety of positive interventions have been developed, which have generally been found to be helpful (Tarragona, 2015). Below is a list of some of the exercises that the positive therapist could draw upon:

- Using one's strengths in new ways: e.g., the therapist might use a questionnaire or other means to elicit the person's character strengths. Having done this the client may be asked to visualize a gap, with them standing on one side and their goals on the other. They are asked to reflect on their top strengths and use each to build a bridge across the gap. 'Describe a way in which you could use that strength to get across the gap to connect with your goal'.
- Affirming one's most important values: e.g., the client is asked to consider their most important values – this itself may take some time and should not be rushed – and when completed they are asked to reflect on their choices, goals and aspirations and how they relate to these values, and what they can do differently that will help them connect how they live their lives more closely to their values.
- Meditating on positive feelings toward self and others: e.g., spending time reflecting on their warm feelings towards others and to themselves, developing self-compassion. When people lack compassion for themselves it may be helpful to ask them to think about how they would feel towards a loved one in a similar situation. Generally, people are more compassionate towards others than to themselves and by reflecting on how they are with others they may learn to be kinder to themselves.
- Visualize their ideal future selves: e.g., the client is asked to imagine that everything works out as they wish, to reflect on what that would be like and the steps it would take to get there.
- Writing letters of gratitude: e.g., the client is asked to think of someone to whom they feel grateful and to write a letter expressing how they feel. They may read the letter out in therapy. Or in some cases it may be appropriate to make contact with the recipient of the gratitude and express thanks directly to them.
- Counting one's blessings, or three good things: e.g., the client is asked to write down three things that have gone well that day. Often this exercise is used as a self-help and recommended that people try just before going to sleep.

- Practising optimism: e.g., the client is shown the difference between pessimistic and optimistic thinking (in terms of explanatory style along the dimensions of internality-externality, globality to specificity, and stable to unstable) and learns to practise noticing what they do and being able to shift from pessimism to optimism.
- Performing acts of kindness: e.g., deliberately making the choice to do things for others.
- Practising mindfulness: e.g., using exercises to help the client learn to stay present-focused and attentive to his inner state and outer environment.
- Using stories to make sense of experiences, finding new metaphors for understanding.

Overall, the evidence for such positive interventions is good. A meta-analysis by Sin and Lyubomirsky (2009) showed that positive interventions yielded medium-sized effects for improvement of well-being and alleviation of depressive symptoms – effect sizes similar to those reported in the classic Smith and Glass (1977) meta-analysis of the effect of psychotherapy. As is evident from the above list, positive activities are simple, brief, intentional activities meant to mimic the myriad positive habits of naturally happy people (e.g., thinking gratefully and optimistically, behaving prosocially). These can be self-administered through the use of simple instructions or included as part of group or individual therapy.

Positive psychology has developed a number of self-help exercises and interventions – books, websites, and smartphone apps (Parks, 2015), but consistent with the person-centred ethos, Parks concludes that when using any self-help tool, guidelines such as frequency of usage and number of activities practised should be determined based on what works for the individual, *not* on what has been done in previous research. For example, the widely used counting one's blessings exercise described above, can be modified in ways that seem helpful to the person.

In terms of finding well-being-inducing activities it is important that they relate to the person's intrinsic motivations. As Layous, Sheldon, and Lyubomirsky (2015) write:

> Of course, some activities will be intrinsically more appealing, and will be easier to jump-start – indeed, this is undoubtedly one advantage of selecting an activity that fits one's personality. For example, rather than jogging around the block, a fitness-seeking wilderness-lover might instead choose to run on a trail through the woods, thereby feeling much less initial resistance to beginning the activity. Rather than expressing one's gratitude and appreciation in a diary, a visually-oriented individual might instead choose to express herself through painting and a musical individual might instead choose to write a song. Such choices would enhance the intrinsic appeal of sitting down to engage in the activity. As these examples illustrate, finding intrinsically-motivated activities may be crucial not only for one's ability to initiate the activity, but also, for one's ability to keep doing the activity in the long term. If the activity becomes boring, then the person may stop doing it. (pp. 193–194)

Person-activity fit is important, and we should not assume that any of the commonly researched variables in positive psychology, such as hope, optimism, forgiveness and so on, will always be helpful. In fact, we should also be wary of when these seemingly positive variables could even be harmful. Take 'forgiveness' as an example. Although we might see this as generally desirable, there are situations in which promoting forgiveness could be harmful (e.g., in abusive relationships). Always, context needs to be taken into account.

Ultimately, the therapist who is using positive interventions is concerned to help their client identify what gives them meaning, pleasure and a sense of engagement. As such, Boniwell, Kauffman, and Silberman (2014) suggest it might even be useful for therapists to pose these three process questions:

- What gives you meaning?
- What gives you pleasure?
- What engages you?

Many of the exercises and techniques that I have been discussing are also used by coaches and so for this next section I will consider the similarities and differences between therapy and coaching.

Therapy versus coaching

Positive therapy as I have described it is not deficit-based, nor focused on only the alleviation of symptoms, but rather is grounded in the meta-theoretical stance of person-centred theory that clients have a tendency towards the realization of their potential. As such, the distinction that is often made between therapy and coaching simply does not apply. In terms of one-to-one practice, Carl Rogers introduced the term counselling but he might equally well have used the term coaching, because in person-centred practice these terms are interchangeable (Joseph, 2006).

However, the coaching profession has distinguished itself from psychological interventions that are aimed at fixing, remedying, or healing something that is pathological. As such, coaching distinguishes itself from therapy, which over the past few decades has become an increasingly medicalized profession and perceived as such by the general public. I am not saying it applies to all therapists, but on the whole this has been a general trend as counsellors increasingly work in health care contexts. But those of us who adopt the person-centred approach do not adopt a medicalized view.

As we have seen, therapy, as it was originally envisaged by Carl Rogers, was never aimed at fixing, remedying or healing. The person-centred practitioner adheres to the same philosophical principle of respecting the self-determination of the other, whether they are practising as a coach or as a therapist. Unlike other therapeutic approaches, person-centred practice is not concerned with 'repairing' or 'curing' dysfunctionality, and has never adopted the 'diagnostic' stance of the medical model in which the therapist is the expert. Like coaching, the focus of person-centred counselling has always been to facilitate the self-determination and full functioning of the client.

The development of different terminology, i.e. counselling versus coaching, to describe people at different points on the spectrum of psychological functioning, reflects the pervasive medical model conception that helping people in distress is different from helping people achieve well-being. It must be emphasized that the way in which professional organizations have developed to deal with people at different points on the spectrum ultimately reflects a social construction of human functioning grounded in a medical model and an illness ideology.

From the person-centred perspective there is no boundary between coaching and counselling. Thus, person-centred coaching is the same activity requiring the same theoretical base, the same skills and high level of personal development as required for person-centred counselling. There is no meaningful theoretical distinction from the perspective of the person-centred approach between the process of coaching and that of counselling. In essence both require principled non-directivity within the context of a facilitative relationship.

This is not to say that there are no differences, but the differences are in the content that clients bring rather than in the process of the therapy itself. Specifically, it is likely that there are differences here in the clients' agendas, with therapy clients being more interested in exploring themselves, their past, and their relation to the world with the aim of personal transformation, and coaching clients being more interested in understanding themselves to the extent that it gives them leverage in achieving their specific future-oriented goals. These differences may be apparent in the sort of things that clients will say during their first session about what they are hoping for. And there may be differences in the wider knowledge and skill base of the practitioner and what they can offer to their client in response to their needs.

For the above reasons, an observer may notice differences between person-centred coaching and person-centred counselling in the content brought by clients and any exercises or assessments used, but careful observation will reveal the process in each case to be the same. Quite simply, what terms we use will determine what clients we work with. If the public understanding is that counselling is about looking back in life at what has gone wrong, whereas coaching is about looking forward to what can go right, different people with different issues will be attracted to counselling than to coaching. Thus, although the task of the person-centred counsellor or coach is the same in either case – to stay with the person and to facilitate the person's process of self-determination – at the level of content the sessions would be different, simply because clients are more likely to bring different material to counselling compared to coaching.

On the other hand, it may be that the use of the term coaching provides a forum for clients who are embarrassed to meet with a counsellor. An example is that of police officers offered the opportunity of counselling in the aftermath of a critical incident. Few took up the opportunity. Following the next critical incident they were offered coaching which was taken up. What they were being offered was person-centred in both cases but the term coaching was less stigmatizing than the term counselling. For person-centred practitioners, where the terminology is interchangeable, which term is used is likely to reflect contexts of employment.

Many coaching practitioners describe themselves as using a person-centred approach, and certainly the general ethos of the person-centred approach, that clients are the best experts on themselves, is one that is readily accepted by the coaching community. The person-centred approach refers to a philosophical *approach* to human relationships not a set of techniques.

Conclusion

There are a variety of existing techniques and therapeutic approaches that positive therapists can use. But I would emphasize that this book is not about technique, it is about re-evaluating our fundamental assumptions as therapists, so that we can introduce experiences for clients from a well-articulated philosophical perspective. As Rollo May (1994), one of the founding fathers of existential therapy, writes:

> Our Western tendency has been to believe that *understanding follows technique*; if we get the right technique, then we can penetrate the riddle of the patient, or, as said popularly with amazing perspicacity, we can 'get the other person's number'. The existential approach holds the exact opposite; namely, that *technique follows understanding*. The central task of the therapist is to seek to understand the patient as a being and as being-in-his-world. All technical problems are subordinate to this understanding. Without this understanding, technical facility is at best irrelevant, at worst a method of 'structuralizing' the neurosis. With it, the groundwork is laid for the therapist's being able to help the patient recognize and experience his own existence, and this is the central process of therapy. This does not derogate disciplined technique; it rather puts it into perspective. (p. 77)

My view is that what is important is the meta-theoretical person-centred assumption that the client is their own best expert and the role of the therapist is to facilitate the client's self-determination.

Further reading

Worsley, R. (2009). *Process work in person-centred therapy* (2nd ed.). Basingstoke: Palgrave.
A summary of the case for process direction by one of the leading scholars in the family of the person-centred and experiential approaches.

Layous, K., Sheldon, K. M., & Lyubomirsky, S. (2015). The prospects, pratices, and perscriptions for the pursuit of happiness. In S. Joseph (Ed.), *Positive psychology in practice: Promoting human flourishing in work, health, education and everyday life* (2nd ed.) (pp. 185–205). Hoboken, NJ: Wiley.

A summary of research in positive psychology and how to help people be happier with a discussion of the importance of person-activity fit.

Joseph, S. (2006). Person-centred coaching psychology: A meta-theoretical perspective. *International Coaching Psychology Review, 1*: 47–55.
The paper in which I first set out the notion of person-centred coaching and its relation to person-centred counselling.

Cooper, M., Schmid, P. F., O'Hara, M., & Bohart, A. C. (Eds). (2013). *The handbook of person-centred psychotherapy and counselling* (2nd ed.). Basingstoke: Palgrave.
The field of person-centred therapy has continued to evolve and this is a collection summarizing the most up-to-date scholarship across the family of person-centred experiential therapies.

Chapter 7

Person-centred psychopathology

As we have seen, positive psychology's aim was to put the study of the good things in life on the agenda. Ever since its inception, however, the relationship of positive psychology to the business-as-usual agenda of psychology to find treatments for psychopathology has been a topic for debate. At the outset it has never been suggested that positive psychology should replace the traditional business of seeking to understand and help people manage their problems. As Folkman and Moskowitz (2003) said:

> those who advocate the study of positive aspects of psychology do not intend that it replace concern with its negative aspects. What appears to be an overemphasis may instead be indicative of a catch-up phase for an area that has been underemphasized in recent years. (p. 121)

Such a position seems to imply that positive psychology is an area of study that sits alongside business-as-usual psychology. As Csikszentmihalyi (2003), one of the founders of positive psychology said:

> Basically, we intended to do our best to legitimize the study of positive aspects of human experience in their own right–not just as tools for prevention, coping, health, or some other desirable outcome. We felt that as long as hope, courage, optimism, and joy are viewed simply as useful in reducing pathology, we will never go beyond the homeostatic point of repose and begin to understand those qualities that make life worth living in the first place. (pp. 113–114)

As such many positive psychologists see what they do as sitting alongside the work of clinical psychologists. Whereas these other psychologists are interested in people's problems in living and helping people move from −5 to 0, they as positive psychologists are interested in helping them move from 0 to +5. The aim of this book is different. This chapter will discuss how positive therapy can be concerned with the full spectrum of −5 to +5.

Challenging the illness ideology

In their groundbreaking critical analysis of the philosophical origins of clinical psychology, and their subsequent development of what they describe as an agenda for 'positive clinical psychology', Maddux, Snyder, and Lopez (2004) argued that clinical psychology is defined by its illness ideology. The origins of this illness ideology – which permeates modern clinical psychology – can be traced back to the earliest origins of the discipline, and the influence of Freud following his visit to Clark University in 1909, leading to the ghost in the machine that we previously discussed.

Grounded in the medico-psychiatric historical context, the illness ideology came to permeate clinical psychology, leading it to focus on what is weak and deficient rather than what is strong and healthy. Maddux, et al. (2004) identified three primary ways in which the adoption of the illness ideology determined the remit of clinical psychology. First, it promotes dichotomies between normal and abnormal behaviours, between clinical and non-clinical problems, and between clinical populations and non-clinical populations. Second, it locates human maladjustment inside the person, rather than in the person's interactions with the environment and their encounters with sociocultural values and social institutions. Third, it portrays people who seek help as victims of intrapsychic and biological forces beyond their control, and thus leaves them as passive recipients of an expert's care.

However, positive psychological approaches to clinical psychology reject these assumptions (Maddux, et al., 2004), replacing them with the idea that we should be 1) as concerned with everyday problems in living as much as with the more extreme variants of functioning, 2) the view that clinical problems differ *only in degree*, rather than in kind, from normal problems in living, 3) that psychological disorders are *not* analogous to biological or medical diseases but are reflective of problems in the person's interactions with his or her environment, and that the role of the positive clinical psychologist is to identify human strengths, and 4) promote mental health. The strategies and techniques they use are educational, relational, social and political, not medical interventions.

Positive clinical psychology as discussed by Maddux and colleagues provides a challenge to the medical model, and offers a way forward for therapists who wish to work with their clients in positive therapeutic ways. As Maddux et al. (2004, p. 332) conclude: 'The major change for clinical psychology, however, is not a matter of strategy and tactic, but a matter of vision and mission'.

The person-centred approach can be seen as a form of positive clinical psychology, but one that makes the additional fundamental assumption that people are inherently motivated towards growth and that psychopathology results when this motivation is usurped and thwarted.

Person-centred view

The central thesis of the person-centred approach is a view of human nature in which people have deep-seated innate propensities towards the actualization of their potentialities. The emphasis of the person-centred approach on helping people to achieve their full potential and optimal functioning might lead some to think that it is only for those who are already relatively well-functioning, and that people with more deep-seated issues and psychological problems would be best advised to seek help from more traditional psychological therapists.

The reader will be aware that I have not yet provided an extensive discussion in this book on the various so-called psychiatric disorders. For some it may seem unusual for a book on therapy not to be more concerned with alleviating distress and dysfunction, or not to use the language of the DSM more extensively. The intention is to be able to speak to the depths of human suffering, but from the perspective of the meta-theory of the actualizing tendency rather than the medical model. In that sense person-centred personality theory, which we looked at earlier, offers a way of understanding how problems arise and psychiatric diagnosis. This was the aim of the book I edited with Richard Worsley on *Person-Centred Psychopathology* in which we asked our contributors to use the language of the person-centred approach to explain diagnostic conditions (Joseph & Worsley, 2005a). Since then others have followed in our footsteps and begun to sketch out more comprehensive person-centred approaches to psychiatric disorders, most notably the work of Sanders and Hill (2014) on counselling for depression. In brief they explain depression using Rogers' theory of incongruence between self and experience. Other work that has set out to use person-centred theory in this way is my own work on post-traumatic stress disorder. In organismic valuing theory person-centred theory is used to integrate post-traumatic stress disorder within a positive psychological framework of post-traumatic growth (Joseph & Linley, 2005). I will say more on this in the next chapter.

But first, in this chapter, I want to show in more detail how it is that person-centred theory provides an alternative to the medical model of psychopathology in the way in which we conceptualize and understand people's psychological problems and how it provides a theoretical integration of the positive and the negative. Previously, I described the idea of how conditions of worth thwart the tendency towards actualization leading to self-actualization incongruent with organismic valuing. To illustrate, Rogers (1980) famously told the story of how as a boy he had observed potatoes beginning to sprout in the dark of his parent's basement:

> The actualizing tendency can, of course, be thwarted or warped, but it cannot be destroyed without destroying the organism. I remember that in my boyhood, the bin in which we stored our winter's supply of potatoes was in the basement, several feet below a small window. The conditions were unfavorable, but the potatoes would begin to sprout — pale, white sprouts, so unlike the healthy green shoots they sent up when planted in the soil in the spring. But these sad, spindly sprouts would grow 2 or 3 feet in length as they reached toward the distant light of the window. The sprouts were, in their bizarre, futile growth, a sort of desperate expression of the directional tendency I have been describing. They would never become plants, never mature, never fulfill their real potential. But under the most adverse circumstances, they were striving to become. Life would not give up, even if it could

not flourish. In dealing with clients whose lives have been terribly warped, in working with men and women on the back wards of state hospitals, I often think of those potato sprouts. So unfavorable have been the conditions in which these people have developed that their lives often seem abnormal, twisted, scarcely human. Yet, the directional tendency in them can be trusted. The clue to understanding their behavior is that they are striving, in the only ways that they perceive as available to them, to move toward growth, toward becoming. To healthy persons, the results may seem bizarre and futile, but they are life's desperate attempt to become itself. (p. 118)

The ways in which a person self-actualizes incongruently to their organismic valuing gives rise to a variety of patterns of distressing and dysfunctional experiences and behaviour. These are not unlike the categories in DSM but because the causative element remains the same there is not the need to classify all the different ways as there is no need for differential diagnosis and treatment.

Helping us understand how incongruence gives rise to psychopathology, Warner (2005, 2007) suggests a range of difficult processes that individuals may experience as a result. Processing is a core human capacity grounded in the biological structure of the organism and that develops naturally within optimal early-childhood relationships. Ideally, guided by organismic valuing people are able to experience fully and accurately their feelings and thoughts, but the more organismic valuing is usurped by conditions of worth the less people are able to regulate, keep in awareness, or attend to their experiences. For example, she has described a 'fragile' processing style, in which individuals are not fully able to 'hold' their own experiences in attention and consequently may easily feel violated, threatened and misunderstood by others:

> Clients who have a fragile style of processing tend to experience core issues at very low or high levels of intensity. They tend to have difficulty starting and stopping experiences that are personally significant or emotionally connected. And, they are likely to have difficulty taking in the point of view of another person while remaining in contact with such experiences. I am not talking about moderate levels of emotional distress. I am talking about moments in which the client's consciousness is flooded with experiences whose intensity is hard to control combined with very high levels of vulnerability and shame. In the midst of these experiences the client is unable to take a broader perspective without a sense of personal annihilation. Most people experience fragile process at the most vulnerable edges of their experience. Some people experience fragile process in relation to a large number of personal experiences, so that it affects large parts of their lives.
>
> For example, a client may talk about day-to-day events for most of a therapy hour and only connect with an underlying feeling of grief at the very end with the sense that she could sob forever. At this point it may be exceedingly difficult for the client to stop the session and to go out into the world alone, much less return to work (Warner, 2008, p. 12).

Warner describes other ways of processing, such as difficult, psychotic and dissociative processes, but the point here is to illustrate that although there may be different patterns of distress and dysfunction, they all stem from the same fundamental cause which is incongruence between self and experience. As such person-centred therapy, involving relational depth, can be helpful in all cases in helping people be more in touch with their experiencing, and help them become more congruent.

Integration of the positive and the negative

As discussed in Chapter 1, positive psychology came about in response to the predominant late twentieth-century orientation of mainstream psychology to disease and the medical model. As such, it is entirely understandable that in the early phase of the history of positive psychology, there was the need for an emphasis on what was different about this approach, i.e. the focus on the positive. Even so, right from the beginning of the positive psychology approach there were those who called for an integrative psychology (Sternberg & Grigorenko, 2001) that explicitly spoke to both the negative and the positive aspects of human experience.

However, 15 years on, the pendulum has now swung away from an exclusive focus on the positive, and is resting at the place of a more balanced approach that includes both the positive and negative aspects of human functioning. Positive psychologists are realizing that to study the positive without understanding its relation to the negative is as flawed as studying the negative without taking account of the positive. But we are still far from achieving the ideal balance, and not yet has theoretical integration been achieved. This is exactly what the person-centred approach offers. Person-centred theory provides an underlying meta-theory of personality development and mental health functioning which can inform positive psychological practice.

Person-centred theory hypothesizes that vulnerability to psychological maladjustment arises through the internalization of conditions of worth. Person-centred theory is able to account for a wide range of psychopathology. While the theory is a unitary one, there are enough nuances in how people experience conditions of worth to account for many of the so-called psychiatric disorders.

Even so, there may be certain problems in living which do not result from the internalization of conditions of worth. No one knows for sure where the boundary is between the psychological and the physiological, and for this reason I would caution against the disregard of the body of knowledge built up about the various so-called psychiatric disorders. As person-centred practitioners and theorists it is important to be knowledgeable about other branches of the psychological professions and how others conceptualize the same issues.

Indeed, as discussed earlier, it is valuable for the person-centred therapist to have the widest possible repertoire of scholarly and therapeutic knowledge so that they can be responsive to the client's needs. It is uncritical acceptance and use of the medical model as a therapeutic strategy that I disagree with, not the possibility that other therapeutic exercises or techniques can at times be helpful.

I have already briefly discussed how problems in living are thought to result from the internalization of conditions of worth, which in turn thwart and usurp the actualizing tendency, leading people to use this propensity towards development to self-actualize in a way consistent with their conditions of worth rather than congruently with their actualizing tendency. But can this theory really account for the range of problems people experience? The aim of this chapter is to show that person-centred theory provides a much more comprehensive account of psychopathology than is generally recognized, and how it provides a powerful alternative to the medical model.

As we have seen earlier, person-centred personality theory provides an account of how severe and enduring psychological problems arise when the actualizing tendency is thwarted, distorted or usurped. For some people, this occurs to such a large extent that it would seem hard to imagine anything constructive in the person so driven they seem by destruction. Despite this, however, the theory remains that their behaviour is still the result of their directional tendency towards actualization, but that it has become so distorted (see Wilkins, 2005a).

Thus, the fact that people behave in various ways that might be described as destructive, distressing or dysfunctional is not evidence that falsifies person-centred theory, because the theory does not say, as some critics mistakenly believe, that people are always 'good'. Critics of Rogers' ideas have taken his emphasis on the actualizing tendency as evidence of 'Pollyanna' theorizing. If humans do have an innate ability to know what is important to them and what is essential for a fulfilling life, how is it, they ask, that so many are distressed and dysfunctional? That would indeed be a naïve position. Rather, what person-centred theory proposes is that people have an intrinsic motivation to develop in a constructive social direction, but that this motivation can be thwarted and usurped.

Even so, it may seem hard to grasp that all of the destructive, distressing and dysfunctional behaviours of humans, simply came about through this unitary theory. Maybe, as some would suggest, the assumption that human nature consists of an intrinsic force towards actualization is just wrong. Maybe some people just don't have a tendency towards actualization. I have heard colleagues in clinical psychology take this view, and say that some people are just born 'wired up' differently. Why does it seem easier to understand destructive, distressing and dysfunctional behaviour as the result of biology than as the result of a developmental process shaped by social and cultural factors? I am of the view that critics of person-centred personality theory have misunderstand the subtle and pervasive influence of conditions of worth, and how easily the actualizing tendency can be thwarted, usurped, distorted and thrown off course, and in turn how this leads people to have difficulties in how they make sense of the world and process emotional information.

Person-centred personality theory describes a very subtle developmental process. In my view, it is not the case that the theory is lacking in explanatory power and that we need to look elsewhere for an explanation of extreme human behaviour. Equally, it is not surprising that the person-centred theory is often misunderstood because it offers a radical alternative paradigm to much of the training in clinical and counselling psychology programmes, which adopt the medical model.

Many in the field of clinical and counselling psychology are shocked when I say this, and respond that they don't adopt the medical model. They then go on to say how they don't view psychological problems as biological or genetic. But this is to misunderstand what is meant by the medical model.

The medical model is the idea that the medical practitioner sets out to identify the problem and to prescribe a specific treatment. This is indeed what much of the training in clinical and counselling psychology does. A quick glance through many of the leading text books in the area show that chapters are set out to describe in turn each of the so-called psychiatric disorders, e.g., depression, anxiety, schizophrenia, obsessive compulsions, post-traumatic stress, and so on, with each of the chapters providing an account of the cause and preferred treatments for each. This is the medical model – the idea that there are specific problems requiring specific treatments.

It is called the medical model because the metaphor is to look upon psychological problems in the same way we look upon medical problems. When we go to see the medical practitioner with a broken leg, we don't want them to give us indigestion tablets; we want them to fix our broken leg. We want the appropriate treatment for our specific problem. The idea behind the textbooks in clinical psychology that lay out the chapters by so-called 'disorder' are no different from this – their task is also to ask what is the specific treatment needed for this specific disorder?

The medical model may be appropriate for understanding some aspects of human suffering, but in my view it has become too pervasive and misled most psychologists into believing that all psychological problems are analogous to medical problems. If one was designing for the first time a profession of psychology there would simply be no logical reason to start with the medical metaphor of human suffering instead of the metaphor of the actualizing tendency. Indeed, it would seem more scientific to begin with the more parsimonious unitary theory and only as it is found wanting to develop more complicated explanations for specific conditions.

But let me be clear that in rejecting the medical model, I am not rejecting the idea of human suffering – only one particular view of how human suffering ought to be understood. There is no doubt that psychological problems can become overwhelming in intensity and duration, causing a person to behave in extremely dysfunctional and dangerous ways, and in ways which are unusual for this person, or unusual for the society he or she lives in. As we have seen, such experiences might be described as psychopathology. I am not saying that psychopathology does not exist. Of course it does – the suffering of many people is all too real. The question is about how we understand psychopathology. I believe that we do ourselves a disservice as therapists in too readily adopting the medical model. What person-centred theory says is that these various forms of psychopathology – depression, anxiety and so on – can be understood as ways in which people have developed as a result of their conditions of worth. As such, the majority of psychological problems are essentially the same in the root cause: they are all expressions of incongruence between self and experience, or in the case of post-traumatic stress the breakdown and disorganisation of a self-structure which is incongruent to experience (see Joseph, 2004).

A positive psychology of mental health

Psychopathology, therefore, is a term that I will use to refer to thoughts, feelings and behaviours that stem from our inner incongruence. This is a person-centred definition, and is different to the way in which many people think about psychopathology. As we have seen, mainstream approaches to psychology and psychiatry adopt the Diagnostic and Statistical Manual (DSM) of Mental Disorders (e.g., American Psychiatric Association, 2013), as a way of cataloguing the various ways in which psychopathology is expressed. While person-centred practitioners do not use the DSM because they reject the medical model and the notion of specific treatments for specific disorders, they do not reject the observation that people experience psychological distress in different ways.

Positive psychologists have begun to address this question too. Peterson (2006), for example, has proposed a model for evaluating psychopathology along the spectrum of strengths, instead of symptoms. He proposes that psychological disorders could be considered as absence or exaggeration of strengths. In this way a disorder may result from the absence of a given character strength, but it can also result from its presence in extreme forms. Moving these arguments forward, Rashid (2015b) has listed the symptoms of major psychological disorders in terms of lack or excess of strengths. For example, depression can result, in part, because of lack of hope, optimism and zest, among other variables; whereas a lack of grit and patience can explain aspects of anxiety. Although this is a powerful way of reconceptualizing disorder, it does not challenge the medical model insofar as differential diagnosis and treatment would still be necessary.

Turning to the person-centred approach, which does challenge the necessity of differential diagnosis, one can understand many of the various expressions of distress listed in DSM as stemming from incongruence, and the idiosyncratic conditions of worth experienced by that person. The concept of conditions of worth describes a process through which people's tendency towards constructive development is thwarted, in such a way that their ability to be in contact with their OVP is weakened at the expense of introjection of these rules for living.

The content of conditions of worth will manifest differently for different people. This is not to say that people can articulate easily what their conditions of worth are, so deeply buried are they within us. For some, conditions are inconsistent causing confusion. For others they may be more consistent either for how to be valued or how to avoid rejection. For others there may be a lack of regard altogether. When one considers the myriad ways in which conditions of worth may be introjected it is not difficult to understand how these manifest in various different behaviour patterns characteristic of psychiatric disorders, but all stemming from the single same source of incongruence.

The person-centred approach also raises some other questions about psychopathology. The first of these is that the term psychopathology is used much more broadly and is not a term confined to being used for people whose behaviours are extreme.

Continuity versus discontinuity

Certainly, psychopathology is a term that refers to a range of seemingly very different psychological problems. One of the tasks of modern psychiatry and psychology has been to try and define various forms of psychopathology, and psychiatrists have produced a classification system containing hundreds of so-called psychiatric disorders (the Diagnostic and Statistical Manual of Mental Disorders; American Psychiatric Association, 2013).

Understanding psychopathology in this way aids communication between professionals who adopt the medical model and who need clear-cut definitions of suffering in order to determine the specific causes and treatments. However, just because this is a widely accepted way of understanding psychopathology does not mean that it is necessarily the best way. The classification of psychiatric disorders is controversial and it is very difficult to draw a clear line between the various disorders. There is much overlap between many of the common psychiatric disorders. Furthermore, it is difficult to draw the line between 'normality' and 'abnormality' so as to be able to say where normality ends and abnormality begins. How long does emotional distress or dysfunction have to last, and how severe does it have to be, for it to be considered as psychopathology? In certain situations it would seem to be perfectly normal to be emotionally distressed, for example, when we are anxious in response to some threat or when we are sad in response to some loss. It is not unusual to be anxious before taking an important exam or to feel sadness at the loss of a loved one. But what of someone who always feel nervous when going into new social situations or someone who remains grieving for years after their loss? Would we say that these are examples of psychopathology?

Answers to such questions will often depend on which perspective is taken on the nature of psychological suffering. Certainly, problems in living are widespread and there is a danger if we pathologize what might be normal and natural reactions to the difficulties of life. While in recent years there has been increased interest in this issue as the DSM seems to increasingly pathologize everyday life with each new edition, throughout the history of psychology many scholars have tackled this issue. Nelson-Jones (1984), for example, drew attention to the difficulties experienced by the majority of people and how most of us struggle to be autonomous in how we live.

Before that Maslow (1970) used the term 'psychopathology of the average' to describe most people's level of functioning. It is in this context that I use the term psychopathology in this book. I do not mean the term to refer only to the extremes of human behaviour, although of course at the extremes psychopathology is more evident. When I use the term 'psychopathology', I am referring to all thoughts, feelings and behaviours that stem from incongruence.

Thus, all of us are incongruent, in some ways, at some times, to some greater or lesser extent. Incongruence is not a categorical entity (i.e. present or absent), but rather a continuous one (i.e. present to some greater or lesser extent).

Normality versus abnormality

As already noted, there have always been critics of a psychiatric establishment that makes judgement over normal versus abnormal behaviours. The difficulties in distinguishing 'normal' from 'abnormal' behaviour were highlighted in a classic 1970s study by Rosenhan (1973, 1975). Rosenhan conducted a now famous experiment in a real life situation showing that psychiatrists' diagnoses were influenced by the social context.

Rosenhan's research team of eight 'normal' people visited twelve different mental hospitals saying that they were experiencing auditory hallucinations and hearing voices saying words like 'dull', 'thud', and 'empty'. The twist was that they weren't really hearing voices. This was part of the experiment which was to investigate the validity of psychiatric diagnoses. Although initially they claimed to be hearing voices they then proceeded to answer all the other questions they were asked by the medical staff honestly. Remembering that this was the 1970s when hospitalization was more common, most of Rosenhan's team were admitted to hospital and diagnosed as schizophrenic. Once inside, the task of the research team (now pseudo-patients) was to convince the hospital staff that they were 'sane'. While inside the hospital, the pseudo-patients behaved 'normally' and insisted on their 'sanity'. The pseudo-patients were hospitalized for between 7 to 52 days with an average length of stay of 19 days. When discharged, the members of the research team were diagnosed as schizophrenic in remission. But what was most interesting was that while they were inside, their 'normal' behaviours were perceived by staff as indicating evidence of schizophrenia. Interestingly, however, some of the other patients were able to identify the pseudo-patients as imposters.

The next step in Rosenhan's research was perhaps even more interesting. Rosenhan informed psychiatric hospitals that pseudo-patients would again present themselves at the hospitals over the next few months. This time, however, there were no pseudo-patients. But, around one-fifth of patients admitted during this time were actually identified by staff as being pseudo-patients (Rosenhan, 1975). The studies by Rosenhan are often taken as evidence for how diagnosis is uncertain and can lead to labelling, and how once a label is attached to a person it becomes a self-fulfilling prophecy.

The experiment by Rosenhan raised important questions about who decides, and on what basis, what is 'normal' and what is 'abnormal'. Much work has accumulated telling us that considerations of what is 'normal' and what is 'abnormal' are not value free. Rather, considerations of 'normality' and 'abnormality' are bound up in cultural and historical contexts (see Littlewood & Lipsedge, 1993). For this reason, critics of the medical model of psychopathology have viewed diagnosis of people as suffering from psychiatric disorders as intrinsically harmful. Maslow summed this up in describing the use of words such as 'patient':

> I hate the medical model that they imply because the medical model suggests that the person who comes to the counsellor is a sick person, beset by disease and illness, seeking a cure. Actually, of course, we hope that the counsellor will be the one who helps to foster the self-actualization of people, rather than the one who helps to cure a disease. (1993, p. 49)

Although there have been many previous critics of the medical model as a way of understanding psychopathology (see Sanders, 2005), many more researchers from within the new positive psychology movement are also now beginning to doubt the validity of the medical model for understanding psychological problems (see Hubble & Miller, 2004; Maddux, 2002; Maddux, Snyder, & Lopez, 2004; Yalom, 2001). In a letters page of the house journal of the British Psychological Society, *The Psychologist*, Marzillier (2004) wrote:

> I am interested in the truth. As a psychotherapist I am confronted every day by the knowledge that evidence-based psychotherapy is a myth. Yet all around me others are extolling its virtues. Do I remain silent because the truth is unpalatable? Or because it might lead to the underfunding of psychotherapy in the NHS [British National Health Service] or some other unwanted consequence? In his wise and useful book on psychotherapy Irving Yalom pointed out that 'if we take the DSM diagnostic system too seriously, if we really believe we are carving at the joints of nature, then we may threaten the human, the spontaneous, the creative and uncertain nature of the therapeutic venture'. Psychotherapy is a creative and uncertain business. It should not be reduced to a collection of treatments for mythical illnesses. (Marzillier, 2004, 625–626)

As an alternative to the medical model, the person-centred psychology of Carl Rogers offers an alternative conceptual model based on people's inherent tendency towards actualization. This view of human nature represents a different paradigm to the medical model that underlies much of contemporary clinical psychology.

Applicability of the positive therapy approach

Person-centred personality theory provides an account of psychopathology that is an alternative to the medical model (see Joseph & Worsley, 2005a). It may be that some experiences do represent abnormal and disordered workings of human physiology and cognitive functioning. For example, schizophrenia, bipolar disorders, temporal lobe epilepsy and organic brain diseases may fall within this category. Also, there may be some psychological problems that are best treated with specific interventions. As Seligman and Peterson (2003) note, there may be some clear specific treatments for some specific disorders, such as applied tension for blood and injury phobia, cognitive therapy for panic and exposure for obsessive-compulsive disorder (for a review, see Seligman, 1994). We do need to determine carefully when psychological problems are best understood through the lens of the medical model. But we should not assume that all psychological problems fall under the spotlight of the medical model and require differential treatment with medical, cognitive, or neuropsychological interventions.

When it comes to the majority of forms of psychological suffering and distress, the key implications of the person-centred approach is that the task is to facilitate the client's organismic valuing process. The goals of therapy do not begin and end with the client being symptom-free, as seen through the lens of a DSM diagnosis. Rather, the person-centred therapist, working to facilitate the client's OVP, would adopt a model of psychopathology grounded in the assumption of an innate actu-alizing tendency, and would work with the understanding that this may facilitate well-being. This is because, as already discussed, when one adopts a model based on the concept of congruence rather than a categorical medical model (i.e., we are either 'ill' or 'not ill'), the facilitation of well-being is synonymous with the alleviation of ill-being. Alleviating psychopathology and facilitating well-being is a unitary task – the end point is positive functioning. As Shlien said in a talk originally given in 1956:

> if the skills developed in psychological counselling can release the construc-tive capacities of malfunctioning people so that they become healthier, this same help should be available to healthy people who are less than *fully* func-tioning. If we ever turn towards positive goals of health, we will care less about where the person begins, and more about how to achieve the desired endpoint of the positive goals. (Shlien, 2003b, p. 26)

Research

Psychological scientists are interested in measurement. Sometimes this may be of phenomena based on diagnostic categories, for example, depression, anxiety or post-traumatic stress. Researchers may wish to test whether a particular therapy is effective for a particular so-called 'disorder'. There is plenty of such research going on, but as already discussed, many person-centred theorists are critical of such research because of the doubtful validity of the DSM system on which the categories of disorder are based. However, others in the person-centred com-munity argue that even if this is the case such research is necessary to maintain their foothold in an increasingly resource-competitive health service in which it is assumed that specific conditions require specific interventions.

I have come to value the ideas inherent in person-centred psychology, but I am aware that if it is to be taken seriously there needs to be supportive research evidence. It will benefit the person-centred movement to produce good quality research that shows that person-centred therapy is effective in the treatment of the various so-called psychiatric disorders.

However, research is not confined to DSM-derived constructs. There are numerous other constructs arising from person-centred theory that can equally well form the basis of research, for example, locus of evaluation, congruence, authenticity, conditions of worth; these can all be measured and their relationships to other variables tested statistically in exactly the same way as researchers have tested constructs from the medical model.

Similarly, self-determination theory, as we have seen, has already provided a wealth of evidence for autonomy, competence, relatedness and their relation to well-being. The constructs we choose to investigate depend on our research question. Carl Rogers was known to say that the facts are always friendly, and by this he did not mean that research was to be used to justify ourselves and our opinions, but rather that we should go with what data tell us, developing our theories in the light of our observations and findings, constantly checking what we think against the scientific evidence. As such I am eager to promote the research agenda into the person-centred approach.

The first step in my view is to reconsider what tools we use to measure therapeutic processes and outcomes. As indicated above, it may be useful politically to use tools that speak to the agenda of DSM in order to provide evidence for person-centred therapy in relation to the various so-called psychiatric disorders, but what is also needed is new research using measures consistent with person-centred theory and positive psychology, a topic I will turn to in Chapter 9.

Conclusion

As we have seen, many positive psychologists reject the categorical approach to psychopathology that is current within clinical psychology and psychiatry. An alternative is person-centred personality theory which, as we have seen, accounts for both psychopathology and well-being through its premise that psychopathology stems from incongruence, i.e. the extent to which people are not acting in accord with their OVP. Well-being arises because people are organismically valuing in their choices and behaviours. Further, we have shown that person-centred personality theory is also entirely consistent, if not fully synonymous, with the assumptions of positive clinical psychology. Person-centred psychology provides a natural continuum that accounts for the varying extents of human experience of psychopathology and well-being, hence, the categorical distinction between positive and negative is viewed as inappropriate, since they are both part of the same vein of human experience.

There is much debate by person-centred practitioners about the use of diagnosis and assessment, and one can understand this debate, given that their position is that there is no need for diagnosis, because there is no need to determine a specific treatment. This is because the actualizing tendency is an alternative paradigm to the medical model. Psychological problems are seen as resulting from the thwarting of the tendency towards actualization, and the nature of each person's psychological problems can be understood when we know more about their developmental social-environmental conditions and the values and beliefs that they have internalized. The actualizing tendency provides a holistic framework that simultaneously spans psychopathology and well-being. In facilitating the actualizing tendency, the therapist is both alleviating psychopathology and promoting well-being.

Further reading

Joseph, S., & Worsley, R. (Eds). (2005a). *Person-centred psychopathology: A positive psychology of mental health*. Ross-on-Wye: PCCS Books.
A collection of renowned person-centred scholars reconceptualize their work in relation to psychiatric diagnosis categories and contemporary issues, in order to engage with mainstream psychology and psychiatry. This book was a landmark in showing there was an alternative way of understanding psychopathology to the medical model.

Sanders, P., & Hill, A. (2014). *Counselling for depression*. London: Sage.
A book underpinned by person-centred theory showing how the person-centred approach can be used to work with depression.

Maddux, J. E., & Lopez, S. J. (2015). Deconstructing the illness ideology and constructing an ideology of human strengths and potential in clinical psychology. In S. Joseph (Ed.), *Positive psychology in practice: Promoting human flourishing in work, health, education and everyday life* (2nd ed.) (pp. 411–427). Hoboken, NJ: Wiley.
A critique of the illness ideology by two of the leading scholars in positive psychology and their views on how to develop new approaches.

Chapter 8

Post-traumatic growth

For the past 20 years much of my own research programme has been concerned with how people respond to trauma. Surprisingly it is the topic of psychological trauma that best illustrates the natural synergy between positive psychology and the person-centred approach. I say surprising because at first glance the topic of trauma is not usually associated with positive psychology. There is so much evidence that traumatic events can precipitate various psychological problems, including depression, anxiety, psychosis and, of course, symptoms of post-traumatic stress (Joseph, Williams, & Yule, 1997). However, more recently there has been much interest in the topic of post-traumatic growth.

Post-traumatic growth is the idea that trauma can often be a transformational force for positive change. The aim of this chapter is to provide a positive therapy view of trauma. A further aim is to illustrate the discussion in the previous chapter about the integration of the positive and the negative by showing how post-traumatic stress can be considered the process by which post-traumatic growth arises.

Defining post-traumatic growth

A number of philosophies and literatures throughout human history have conveyed the idea that there is personal gain to be found in suffering. The observation that traumatic events can provoke positive psychological changes is also contained in the major religions of Buddhism, Christianity, Hinduism, Islam and Judaism. Within humanistic and existential philosophy and psychology it has also long been recognized that positive changes can come about as a result of suffering (e.g. Frankl, 1963; Jaffe, 1985; Kessler, 1987). For example, serious illness is often a trigger for growth, and the application of positive therapy to health psychology seems particularly relevant, particularly within the context of life-threatening illness, such as cancer. As Yalom writes:

> A real confrontation with death usually causes one to question with real seriousness the goals and conduct of one's life up to then. So also with those who confront death through a fatal illness. How many people have lamented: 'what a pity I had to wait till now, when my body is riddled with cancer, to know how to live!' (1989, p. 26)

The observation that stressful and traumatic events could provide opportunities for positive reappraisal and personal growth was also noted in the 1980s by scholars in stress and coping (e.g., Antonovsky, 1987; Lazarus & Folkman, 1984; Taylor, 1983). It began to be noted in the post-traumatic stress literature in the early 1990s (e.g., Herman, 1992; Janoff-Bulman, 1992; Joseph, Williams, & Yule, 1993; Lyons, 1991; Snape, 1997), becoming a topic of study in its own right in late 1990s (O'Leary & Ickovics, 1995; Tedeschi, Park, & Calhoun, 1998a). Now, almost 20 years later it is an established field of study and one of the flagship topics of positive psychology (Joseph, 2011).

Various terms have been used to describe the constellation of positive changes often reported by people following stressful and traumatic events (Linley & Joseph, 2004b), such as construing benefits (Affleck & Tennen, 1996), perceived benefits (McMillen & Fisher, 1998), stress-related growth (Armeli, Gunthert, & Cohen, 2001; Park, 1998; Park, Cohen, & Murch, 1996), transformational coping (Aldwin, 1994), and thriving (Abraido-Lanza, Guier, & Colon, 1998). The most popular term is that of post-traumatic growth introduced by the pioneering scholars and clinicians Richard Tedeschi and Lawrence Calhoun (Tedeschi & Calhoun, 1995, 1996).

Since post-traumatic stress disorder (PTSD) is described within the DSM, there may be a misperception that for growth to occur, one must be traumatized as defined by a diagnosis of PTSD. The term post-traumatic growth, however, is not anchored to PTSD. People can experience post-traumatic growth whether or not they have had a previous diagnosis of PTSD. Tedeschi and Calhoun have emphasized this point in several of their writings that the events that precede growth do not necessarily need to be traumatic in the sense of the DSM (Tedeschi, Park, & Calhoun, 1998b).

Post-traumatic growth has three main facets. First, people often report that their relationships are enhanced in some way, for example that they now value their friends and family more, and feel an increased compassion and altruism toward others. Second, survivors change their views of themselves in some way, for example, that they have a greater sense of personal resiliency, wisdom and strength, perhaps coupled with a greater acceptance of their vulnerabilities and limitations. Third, there are often reports of changes in life philosophy, for example, survivors report finding a fresh appreciation for each new day, and renegotiating what really matters to them in the full realization that their life is finite (see Joseph, 2011). For some, there is also a religious or spiritual component to their changes in life philosophy (Calhoun, Cann, Tedeschi, & McMillan, 2000: Koenig, Pargament, & Nielsen, 1998; Shaw, Joseph, & Linley, 2005).

These positive changes in psychological well-being can underpin a whole new way of living. People may learn to appreciate each day to the full, believe themselves to be wiser or act more altruistically in the service of others, and may dedicate their energies to social renewal or political activism. There is a shift from the self-perception of oneself as a victim to a survivor and even to being a thriver (Joseph, 2011). Such trauma survivors embrace their newfound positive approach to life within a context of tragic hopefulness. They know first-hand the ups and downs, and the limits of human life. This awareness guides them to live their lives in a way that is truly and positively authentic, interpreting their trauma as a valued learning opportunity and giving back to others through the benefit of their experience.

Measurement of post-traumatic growth

Several self-report psychometric tools have been developed to assess personal growth and positive change following adversity. The first such measure to be developed was the Changes in Outlook Questionnaire (CiOQ) developed by Joseph, Williams, and Yule (1993) (see Table 8.1). The CiOQ provides a self-report assessment, in keeping with positive psychology, of the extent to which a person has experienced both positive changes and negative changes following adversity and trauma. The CiOQ consists of 26 items, 11 assess positive changes and 15 assess negative changes. The 11 positive items are summed to give a total score ranging from 11 to 66. The 15 negative items are summed to give a total score ranging from 15 to 90.

Since the CiOQ was first developed extensive work into the psychometric properties of the CiOQ has been carried out confirming its reliability and validity (see Joseph et al., 2005). My students and I have also used it in a number of studies, documenting changes in people following, for example, the events of September 11th, 2001 (Linley et al., 2003) and in therapists who work with distressed people following trauma (Linley et al., 2005). In one study, it was used to assess positive changes in patients undergoing treatment for cancer. A large percentage of patients endorsed positive changes. The change that was most agreed with was that of valuing relationships much more now, followed by not taking life for granted anymore (see Martin, Tolosa, & Joseph, 2004) (see Table 8.2).

The CiOQ promises to be a useful tool when working with clients who have experienced trauma and adversity. For practitioners who may need brief and quick-to-administer measures we have also developed a short version of the CiOQ (Joseph et al., 2006).

Several other self-report psychometric tools were also published during the 1990s to assess positive changes following trauma, notably the *Posttraumatic Growth Inventory* (PTGI; Tedeschi & Calhoun, 1996); the *Stress-Related Growth Scale* (SRGS; Park, Cohen, & Murch, 1996), the *Perceived Benefit Scale* (PBS; McMillen & Fisher, 1998), and the *Thriving Scale* (TS; Abraido-Lanza, Guier, & Colon, 1998).

The newest tool for the assessment of growth following adversity is the Psychological Well-Being–Post-Traumatic Changes Questionnaire (PWB–PTCQ: Joseph, Maltby, Stockton, Hunt, & Regal, 2012). This measure reframes the concept of growth following adversity as an increase in psychological well-being (PWB) as opposed to subjective well-being (SWB) (Joseph & Linley, 2008b). As we have seen earlier, SWB can be broadly defined as emotional states whereas PWB refers to high levels of autonomy, environmental mastery, positive relations with others, openness to personal growth, purpose in life and self-acceptance within contemporary literature (see Ryff & Singer, 1996). Based on

Table 8.1 Changes in Outlook Questionnaire (CiOQ)

Each of the following statements were made by people who experienced stressful and traumatic events in their lives about how the event had changed them. Thinking about how you have changed since the event, please read each one and indicate, by circling the number, how much you agree or disagree with it AT THE PRESENT TIME.

1 = Strongly disagree, 2 = Disagree, 3 = Disagree a little, 4 = Agree a little, 5 = Agree, 6 = Strongly agree.

		Strongly disagree	Disagree	Disagree a little	Agree a little	Agree	Strongly agree
1	I don't look forward to the future anymore.	1	2	3	4	5	6
2	My life has no meaning anymore.	1	2	3	4	5	6
3	I no longer feel able to cope with things.	1	2	3	4	5	6
4	I don't take life for granted anymore.	1	2	3	4	5	6
5	I value my relationships much more now.	1	2	3	4	5	6
6	I feel more experienced about life now.	1	2	3	4	5	6
7	I don't worry about death at all anymore.	1	2	3	4	5	6
8	I live everyday to the full now.	1	2	3	4	5	6
9	I fear death very much now.	1	2	3	4	5	6
10	I look upon each day as a bonus.	1	2	3	4	5	6
11	I feel as if something bad is just waiting around the corner to happen.	1	2	3	4	5	6
12	I'm a more understanding and tolerant person now.	1	2	3	4	5	6
13	I have a greater faith in human nature now.	1	2	3	4	5	6
14	I no longer take people or things for granted.	1	2	3	4	5	6

Table 8.1 (Continued)

	Strongly disagree	Disagree	Disagree a little	Agree a little	Agree	Strongly agree
15	I desperately wish I could turn the clock back to before it happened.	1	2	3	4	5	6
16	I sometimes think it's not worth being a good person.	1	2	3	4	5	6
17	I have very little trust in other people now.	1	2	3	4	5	6
18	I feel very much as if I'm in limbo.	1	2	3	4	5	6
19	I have very little trust in myself now.	1	2	3	4	5	6
20	I feel harder towards other people.	1	2	3	4	5	6
21	I am less tolerant of others now.	1	2	3	4	5	6
22	I am much less able to communicate with other people.	1	2	3	4	5	6
23	I value other people more now.	1	2	3	4	5	6
24	I am more determined to succeed in life now.	1	2	3	4	5	6
25	Nothing makes me happy anymore.	1	2	3	4	5	6
26	I feel as if I'm dead from the neck downwards.	1	2	3	4	5	6

NB: items 4, 5, 6, 7, 8, 10, 12, 13, 14, 23 and 24 are summated to give a total score for the positive response scale (CiOP). Items 1, 2, 3, 9, 11, 15, 16, 17, 18, 19, 20, 21, 22, 25 and 26 are summated to give a total score for the negative response scale (CiON).

Table 8.2 Percentage of respondents (n = 76) following cancer treatment agreeing with
each of the statements on the Changes in Outlook Questionnaire Positive
Scale (see Martin et al., 2004)

	% Strongly agreed	% Agreed	% Agreed a little
I value my relationships much more now.	53	35	9
I don't take life for granted any more.	47	39	8
I feel more experienced about life now.	39	38	18
I no longer take people or things for granted.	37	39	16
I live every day to the full now.	36	41	14
I look upon each day as a bonus.	45	26	17
I value other people more now.	32	41	15
I am more determined to succeed in life now.	37	25	21
I'm a more understanding and tolerant person now.	18	26	30
I have greater faith in human nature now.	12	23	36
I don't worry about death at all any more.	18	12	23

this conceptualization the PWB–PTCQ is an 18 item self-report tool for assessing
change following adversity and trauma (see Table 9.4, Chapter 9).

How common is post-traumatic growth?

Each of these measures, like the CiOQ, asks respondents to think about how they
have changed since an event and to rate the extent of their change on a series of
items. Using such measures of perceived growth, and open-ended interviews, a
large number of studies have shown that growth is common for survivors of various
traumatic events, including transportation accidents (shipping disasters, plane
crashes, car accidents), natural disasters (hurricanes, earthquakes), interpersonal
experiences (combat, rape, sexual assault, child abuse), medical problems (cancer, heart attack, brain injury, spinal cord injury, HIV/AIDS, leukaemia, rheumatoid arthritis, multiple sclerosis, illness) and other life experiences (relationship
breakdown, parental divorce, bereavement, immigration). Typically 30–70 per
cent of survivors will say that they have experienced positive changes of one form
or another (Linley & Joseph, 2004b; Prati & Pietrantoni, 2009).

What factors are associated with post-traumatic growth?

Numerous studies show that problem-focused and emotion-focused coping
strategies are related to growth. Prati and Pietrantoni (2009), who conducted a
meta-analysis of 103 studies showing that optimism, social support, spirituality,
acceptance coping, reappraisal coping, religious coping and seeking social support were associated with post-traumatic growth.

Practitioners in health, clinical and counselling psychology will encounter patients daily whose lives have been affected by such events. Up to now practitioners may have drawn on theories of post-traumatic stress to help their patients. Positive therapy involves a shift in perception from the medical model to the person-centred approach, in which we begin to understand that growth is the normal and natural motivation of people following trauma (Joseph, 2011). In the following section, I will describe how person-centred theory can be developed to understand response to traumatic events. Specifically, I will describe the organismic valuing theory (Joseph & Linley, 2005).

Organismic valuing and post-traumatic growth

Research is now untangling a seemingly intricate dance between post-traumatic stress processes and post-traumatic growth. The most successful attempt to date is organismic valuing theory which explains how post-traumatic growth arises as a result of post-traumatic stress. This is a person-centred theory because at its core is the theoretical assumption that people are intrinsically motivated towards growth, and that this will result in greater eudaimonic functioning. However, such growth is not automatic but requires the right social environment. Organismic theory draws together information processing and social cognitive theories of post-traumatic stress with research on self-determination theory to show how trauma leads to a breakdown in self-structure, signalled by the experiences of post-traumatic stress indicating the need to cognitive-process the new trauma-related information (Joseph & Linley, 2005).

The characteristics of post-traumatic growth described above have long been of interest to person-centred psychologists. What we now call post-traumatic growth might be viewed in terms of a movement toward becoming what Rogers (1959) referred to as fully functioning (see Joseph, 2003b, 2004, 2005). As discussed in Chapter 3, the fully functioning person is someone who is accepting of themselves; values all aspects of themselves – their strengths and their weaknesses; is able to live fully in the present; experiences life as a process; finds purpose and meaning in life; desires authenticity in themselves, others, and societal organizations; values deep trusting relationships; is compassionate towards others, and able to receive compassion from others; and is acceptant that change is necessary and inevitable.

The characteristics of the fully functioning person are synonymous with those of post-traumatic growth. As with descriptions of post-traumatic growth, the description of the fully functioning person is primarily a description of the development of psychological well-being rather than subjective well-being (see also Chapter 2).

As we have seen, what Rogers (1959) proposed was that individuals have an innate tendency towards actualization of their potentialities, and when individuals are provided with a facilitative social environment they will actualize towards becoming fully functioning. In the person-centred psychology of Rogers, the social environment necessary to facilitate this innate tendency towards actualization is one characterized by, among other things, unconditional positive regard.

In brief, Rogers hypothesized that when people feel themselves to be unconditionally accepted, they do not feel the need to be defensive. As such they drop their psychological defences which permits them to be able to realistically appraise the person-environment interaction. Through realistic appraisal processes, people are able to move psychologically towards becoming fully functioning. As we have seen in Chapter 4, evidence suggests that people grow when there is contact with the organismic valuing process.

I would argue that individuals have innate developmental trends and propensities towards growth that may be given voice by an organismic valuing process occurring within them. A person-centred perspective on trauma emphasizes that growth is the natural endpoint of trauma resolution (Joseph, 2003b, 2004, 2005; see also Christopher, 2004).

Shattered assumptions

The confrontation with an adverse event has a shattering effect on the person's assumptive world. Traumatic events show us that we are fragile, that the future is uncertain and that life is not just. Traumatic events show us the limits of the human condition and bring into question our assumptions about ourselves and the world (Janoff-Bulman, 1989, 1992). The phenomenology of post-traumatic stress disorder (PTSD), the states of intrusion and avoidance, according to Horowitz (1982, 1986) and Janoff-Bulman (1992) are indicative of the need to cognitively and emotionally process the new trauma-related information and to rebuild a new assumptive world.

As Creamer et al. (1992) argue, the symptoms of PTSD are indicative of network resolution processing, and the fact that the person is cognitively engaged in trying to work through their experience. Individual differences in trauma response are explained in organismic valuing process theory in terms of the degree of disparity between the trauma and pre-existing expectations and beliefs.

Recovery from trauma in these theoretical perspectives is explained as resulting from either assimilation of the traumatic memory or a revision of existing schemas to cognitively accommodate new information. Organismic valuing process theory holds that it is human nature to rebuild a new assumptive world that positively accommodates the new trauma-related information. That is to say, people are intrinsically motivated to find meaning in and seek benefit from their experience and the natural end point of trauma resolution is growth. But this does not always happen, unless the social environment provides the basic nutrients for growth.

Accommodation versus assimilation

Thus, organismic theory posits that human beings are active, growth-oriented organisms. People are naturally inclined to cognitively accommodate their psychological experiences into a unified sense of self and a realistic view of the world. The process of cognitive accommodation is such that the person's assumptive world is rebuilt in light of their experiences. This is in contrast to the process of cognitive assimilation where the person appraises their experiences in such a way as to be consistent with their assumptive world. Growth, by definition, requires accommodation rather than assimilation.

However, although the theory says that people are intrinsically motivated towards accommodation, the theory also posits that extrinsic social-environmental forces can usurp this process leading the person to assimilate rather than accommodate. For example, within the social psychology literature there is much work on how victims will often self-blame inappropriately in order to maintain their sense of the world as just and controllable (see Joseph, 1999). If an event happens which seems to be for no reason this can be unsettling, and so people sometimes cope with such events by perceiving themselves as to blame which although providing an explanation for what happened which is more settling, is obviously unhelpful in other ways.

How we make sense of the world is of course influenced by the people around us. Other people influence our appraisal processes, and can therefore say and do things which will either facilitate or impede the process of accommodation. In the above example, perhaps others are unsettled too, and in their attempts to be supportive inadvertently encourage us to self-blame, impeding the process of accommodation, and leading us to assimilate our experience. If we were to accommodate our experience, we would rebuild our world view to acknowledge that events are sometimes random and strike us for no good reason. This might be unsettling but it is true. To assimilate the experience means to defend ourselves from this truth.

As such, post-traumatic growth involves the rebuilding of the shattered assumptive world. This can be illustrated through the metaphor of the shattered vase (see Joseph, 2011). Imagine that one day you accidentally knock a treasured vase off its perch. It smashes into tiny pieces. What do you do? Do you try to put the vase back together as it was? Do you collect the pieces and drop them in the rubbish, as the vase is a total loss? Or do you pick up the beautiful coloured pieces and use them to make something new – such as a colourful mosaic? When adversity strikes, people often feel that at least some part of them – be it their views of the world, their sense of themselves, their relationships – has been smashed. Those who try to put their lives back together exactly as they were remain fractured and vulnerable. But those who accept the breakage and build themselves anew become more resilient and open to new ways of living.

Meaning as comprehension versus meaning as significance

Thus, the organismic valuing theory of growth through adversity posits an intrinsic motivation towards cognitive accommodation of the new trauma-related information. Accommodation requires a shift in meaning, of which two kinds can be delineated, a shift in meaning as comprehension, and shift in meaning as significance (e.g., Davis, Nolen-Hoeksema, & Larson, 1998; Janoff-Bulman & Frantz, 1997). Cognitive accommodation processes require changes in meaning as significance, and this can be in either a negative or a positive direction. A person can accommodate new trauma-related information, for example, that random events happen in the world and that bad things can happen at any time, in one of two ways. This accommodation may be made in a negative direction (e.g., a depressogenic reaction of hopelessness and helplessness), or in a positive direction of meaning as significance (e.g., that life is to be lived more in the here and now). It is thought that it is human nature to be intrinsically motivated towards a positive accommodation of the new trauma-related information as opposed to a negative accommodation, insofar as an evolutionary psychology approach would suggest that this should be more adaptive. As Christopher (2004) pointed out, in describing a theory that extensively fills out the biological aspects of reactions to trauma, from an evolutionary point of view trauma breaks up culturally acquired attitudes and creates the possibility of new meanings and more adaptive responses to the environment.

Three cognitive outcomes

In this theory, the states of intrusion and avoidance characteristic of PTSD are indicative of cognitive-emotional processing and the need to rebuild the assumptive world. Thus, PTSD will diminish to the extent that the new trauma-related information is either accommodated or assimilated. As the person begins to either accommodate or assimilate their experience, three possible cognitive outcomes to the psychological resolution of trauma-related difficulties are therefore posited. First, experiences may be assimilated (i.e., return to pre-trauma baseline). Second, that experiences may be accommodated in a negative direction. Third, experiences may be accommodated in a positive direction.

The possibility of the three cognitive outcomes helps to resolve the question of why it is that previously traumatized people often appear to be more vulnerable rather than more resistant to the effects of future stressful and traumatic events. Attempts at assimilation rather than accommodation are common. People who assimilate their experience thus maintain their pre-event assumptions despite the evidence to the contrary, and thus would be expected to develop more rigid defences, which in turn leaves them with increased vulnerability for future development of post-traumatic stress.

It may be hypothesized that the alleviation of post-traumatic stress may come about through either assimilation or accommodation processes, but by definition only accommodation can be 'growthful' as it involves change. But accommodation is in itself not necessarily positive as the new trauma-related information can be accommodated either negatively or positively. What determines the direction of accommodation is the extent to which the person is able to organismically evaluate their experiences, and to find the appropriate rebalance of their assumptive world.

In summary, what the organismic valuing process theory posits is that the person is intrinsically motivated towards the rebuilding of an assumptive world in a direction consistent with the new trauma-related information. This leads to greater psychological well-being, although not necessarily greater subjective well-being. The theory holds that this occurs when the social environment is able to meet the individual's needs for autonomy, competence and relatedness, then the organismic valuing process is promoted.

First, organismic valuing process theory is first and foremost a theory of psychological well-being. Second, organismic valuing process theory is consistent with the notion of an underlying completion principle, but extends this concept so that the completion principle is viewed as an expression of part of the tendency towards actualization. Third, organismic valuing theory is consistent with the notion that accommodation rather than assimilation is necessary for growth. Fourth, organismic valuing process theory is consistent with the notion that it is meaning as significance that underlies growth rather than meaning as comprehensibility.

What the organismic valuing process theory posits is that the person is intrinsically motivated towards the rebuilding of the assumptive world in a direction consistent with their innate propensities toward actualization of the potentialities. As part of this innate process the individual is motivated to engage in a realistic reappraisal of the meaning of the event and its existential implications. This leads to greater psychological well-being. For most, post-traumatic growth is a process that unfolds gradually over a period of time as the person cognitively accommodates the new trauma-related material.

Organismic valuing refers to how intrinsic motivation is experienced by the person. One woman who was caught up in a fatal shooting in which her close friend was killed and who had suffered from considerable post-traumatic stress for several years said how she woke early one morning after a night of restless sleep and got up to look at a picture of her children.

> In the silent wee hours of the morning, I sat staring at their picture and began to sob. Through my sobs, I heard the real voice of wisdom I believe we all possess. It was my voice, the voice that knows me best, but a voice that had become muted. Guess what. No one is coming to change the situation. No one will rescue you. No one can. It's up to you. Find your strength. I realized that as long as I remained a victim, I too made my family a victim. My anxiety could only teach them to be anxious. I was robbing them of happiness and a positive outlook on the world. I had come to the intersection of intersections. I could choose to end my life or 'I could choose to live. I needed to live for my family – and later I understood most importantly, for myself.' (quoted in Joseph, 2012, p. 142)

Organismic valuing process theory suggests that what is paramount in facilitating growth after adversity is helping the client to hear their own inner voice of wisdom and to articulate their own inner experiencing, and thus to accommodate the new trauma-related information rather than assimilate it.

The implication of organismic valuing process theory is that the therapist can help their client to accommodate the new trauma-related information. The theory suggests that a therapist who is authentic, empathic and listens unconditionally to the client, helping them to more clearly articulate the new meanings as they begin to emerge, will facilitate the client's organismic valuing process, and thus their accommodation of the new trauma-related information in a positive direction.

In contrast, a therapist whose style of working more reflects their own values or other social conventions might serve to push the client towards assimilation of the trauma-related information. Assimilation would involve trying to comprehend the event in such a way as to maintain the prior assumptions about the self and the world. For example, some events threaten our self-esteem. As a result, we may be motivated to blame others because by blaming others we can say to ourselves that we were not to blame. As such we are able to maintain our self-esteem. As already mentioned, other events threaten our sense of justice. In order to preserve a sense of justice we may be motivated to blame ourselves. By blaming ourselves we are able to maintain a belief in a world in which we get what we deserve. As such justice is preserved. These are the costs and benefits of blame and how it can be used to help assimilate the new trauma-related information (Joseph, 1999). But of course, while we may be seeking to maintain certain assumptions by using blame, inevitably we have to live with the discomfort of these cognitive strategies.

Facilitating post-traumatic growth

There are different ways in which therapists can support the basic needs of clients and follow their direction, and our understanding of how to do this is enhanced when we have a view of the general psychological processes involved in recovery and growth following adversity. The main implication of the organismic valuing theory is that the task of the therapist is to provide a social environment that is able to support the continuous cycle of processing, on the understanding that when blocks are removed affective-cognitive processing will follow (see Joseph, Murphy, & Regal, 2012).

In Chapter 6, I discussed the notion of process direction and the facilitation of post-traumatic growth provides a good example of the ways in which survivors might express needs that the therapist can respond to by introducing experiences into the session.

1   Clients may talk about social support processes that may be impeding processing, e.g., friends and family not being supportive in ways that the client would like. The therapist might make suggestions on obtaining other forms of support or how to elicit the desired forms of support more effectively.
2   Clients may begin to talk about events in way that shows they recognize a need within them to confront their memories. The therapist might suggest

engaging in exposure-related activities to promote reappraisal of the traumatic experience and its meanings. By exposure I mean any activities that allow for confrontation of the trauma-related information in a safe controlled environment; this includes talking and listening to structured exposure-based exercises. It may also involve actively engaging in the physical act of accompanying the client in a feared situation and supporting them through the experience, teaching them how to re-interpret environmental stimuli they have learned to be fearful of.

3   Clients might talk about feeling that they are going mad. It may be appropriate to facilitate reappraisal of the emotional states to which such appraisals give rise, perhaps by discussing the nature of PTSD, thus helping to normalize distressing emotional states, for example.

4   Clients might talk about now being able to cope. The therapist could promote helpful coping strategies: supporting developing new coping skills, strategies for seeking social support, safe place imagery, for example.

5   The client may appear in a high state of distress, saying that they wish they felt calmer. The therapist may reduce negative emotional states and promote positive emotional states: relaxation exercises, gratitude exercises, for example.

Conclusion

In this chapter a person-centred account of adaptation to trauma is described. In essence, this theory proposes that when people's basic psychological needs for autonomy, competence and relatedness are met through a supportive social environment, then their organismic valuing process will be facilitated, and they will be able to accommodate positively the new trauma material, changing their views and perceptions in light of this new information. This positive accommodation leads to increases in psychological well-being, but not necessarily increases in subjective well-being, as the person rebuilds their assumptive world in a way that is more congruent with their organismic valuing process. These increases in psychological well-being are characterized as post-traumatic growth, and also represent a movement towards becoming more fully functioning.

A fundamental element of this process is the role of the therapist, since the OVP theory of growth posits that the therapist should only work to facilitate the OVP of the client, and should not allow the therapy to be driven by the therapist's own agenda, values or beliefs. The danger of the therapist leading the therapy encounter, rather than facilitating the client's OVP, is that the client could be led to assimilate the trauma material, thus leaving them vulnerable in the future. Further research is needed to test and elaborate the various aspects of both the organismic valuing theory of growth and the principles of positive therapy more broadly.

Further reading

Tedeschi, R. G., & Calhoun, L. G. (1996). The posttraumatic growth inventory: Measuring the positive legacy of trauma. *Journal of Traumatic Stress, 9*, 455–471.
The paper that caught the imagination and introduced the world to post-traumatic growth.

Joseph, S. (2004). Client-centred therapy, post-traumatic stress, and post-traumatic growth: Theoretical perspectives and practical implications. *Psychology and Psychotherapy: Theory, Research and Practice, 77*, 101–120.
The first paper to explicitly use Rogers' theory to integrate the ideas of PTSD and post-traumatic growth within a single framework, with a set of action points for research and practice.

Joseph, S. (2011). *What doesn't kill us: The new psychology of posttraumatic growth*. New York: Basic Books.
Overview and summary of the field of post-traumatic growth introducing the metaphor of the shattered vase.

Chapter 9

Theoretically consistent measurement

The aim of this chapter is to discuss the use of measurement within positive therapy. The advent of positive psychology has challenged the traditional focus on psychiatric categories to redefine the goals of therapy. Today, we can look to the concepts of well-being, human flourishing and happiness. There is now a need to develop research into the effectiveness of therapy for the promotion of positive psychological outcomes and processes. For research purposes in clinical settings, the therapist may want the client to complete questionnaires at regular intervals over the course of therapy, in order to gather evidence that their work is effective. An organization may wish to gather such data from a number of workers in order to provide evidence for what their organization is able to provide.

Positive psychology offers many instruments that can be used in research and also in practice. It may be that the use of such measures can be therapeutic in themselves. What is unusual about these and similar positive psychological measures in contrast to traditionally used measures in therapy is that they are all focused on what the person can do, what their abilities are and what the good things in life are for them. In this sense, positive psychology offers a range of tools that are theoretically consistent with the notion of positive therapy with its emphasis on developing psychological well-being, rather than alleviating distress and dysfunction. Many therapists will welcome these changes and will readily include new measures of positive functioning within their practice, either alongside or as replacements for the traditional measures of psychiatry.

As I have begun to illustrate in the previous chapter on post-traumatic growth, there are many tests and measures in positive psychology that clients may themselves find useful, and which help them understand themselves. In this chapter I will say more about how tests and measures can be used in ways that are supportive of people's directions and may form the focus for collaboration in the therapy or coaching session.

Positive psychology assessment

Positive psychology is still relatively new and although psychologists have many measurement tools at their disposal, most of these are solely concerned with aspects of psychopathology (e.g., Corcoran & Fisher, 2000). There are hundreds of tests available to measure constructs such as anxiety, depression, stress and so on, but over the past decade since the development of the positive psychology perspective there has been an explosion of interest in new measures to assess well-being.

Positive psychology research tells us the importance of helping our clients realize their strengths. One of the debates in therapy is about how we actually go about doing this – how do we help people realize their strengths? The person-centred approach suggests that in a therapeutic relationship in which the client feels valued, accepted and not judged, they will inevitably be drawn to exploring and understanding their strengths. Seen this way, people are motivated towards using their strengths when the hold of their conditions of worth become loosened, and it is the direction towards which clients will take us. We don't need to direct clients towards doing this but it may be helpful to provide our clients with a map of what for many will be uncharted territory.

Strength-based assessment

Strengths-based assessment has been a cornerstone of positive psychology since its inception. As Peterson and Seligman (2004) describe, one's signature strengths convey a sense of ownership and authenticity, an intrinsic yearning to use them, and a feeling of inevitability in doing so. Using one's signature strengths is congruent with one's intrinsic interests and values. In many senses, one can understand Peterson and Seligman's description of strengths here as being representative of what, within person-centred theory, is referred to as the actualizing tendency.

Within a supportive environmental context, the client's strengths will be recognized and become a topic of exploration for them. This does not mean necessarily that they will talk abstractly about their strengths as one would if opening a conversation about using their strengths, but that over the course of therapy it will be the natural direction of travel that clients will be in some way or another discussing using, yearning to use, preparing to think about, how they could better be themselves.

Emphasis on strength-based assessment is consistent with positive therapy. For many therapists this will not have been a standard part of their traditional practice, but as should be evident, strengths-based assessment is widely accepted in humanistic, educational or solution-focused approaches to coaching, and can have a place in therapy. As Rashid (2015b) writes:

> Assessing strengths can provide the clinician with a powerful tool to understand a client's intact repertoires, which can be effectively utilized in treatment planning, enabling clients and clinicians to intervene and evaluate treatment through multiple avenues (reduction in symptoms, increase in positive emotions, improved social relationships, better work-life balance, etc.). Considering what strengths a client brings to effectively deal with troubles stimulates a very different discussion and therapeutic relationship from a deficit-oriented inquiry probing, 'What weaknesses have led to your

symptoms?' Strength-based assessment offers distinct advantages. Assessing strengths changes the orientation of clinical services from remediation to nurturance of resilience and wellbeing. Knowledge of strengths offers clients an additional but important strategy to solve their problems, which likely increases their self-efficacy. Assessment and deployment of strengths such as optimism, hope, zest, curiosity, creativity, social intelligence, and gratitude cultivates positive emotions. (p. 521)

Various measurement tools are available that can be helpful to clients. For example, the Myers-Briggs Type Indicator (MBTI) is a widely used and popular measure. It is an application of Jungian theory widely used, more in coaching than in therapy, but nonetheless it can be helpful because it promotes the notion that all personality types have equal value although they may have different ways of contributing. For example, it is not seen as better to be introverted or extraverted but it is recognized that people with each of these styles have different ways of being in the world.

Various dedicated measures exist with which to assess strengths. The most widely used is the Values in Action (VIA) instrument developed by Peterson & Seligman (2004). The VIA describes twenty-four strengths that divide into six categories: Cognitive, Humanity, Community, Courage, Temperance and Transcendence.

Measures of well-being

In the sections below I will describe some of the measures that my colleagues and I have developed. The aim is not to provide a comprehensive list of measures but to illustrate the different ways in which the ideas of positive psychology can be applied.

Positive functioning inventory

In order to address one measurement need of the applied positive psychologist and positive therapist, the Positive Functioning Inventory (PFI-12: Joseph & Maltby, 2014) is a 12-item self-report questionnaire (see Table 9.1). Six items ask about positive thoughts, feelings and bodily experiences. Six items ask about negative thoughts, feelings and bodily experiences. Respondents are asked to think about how they have felt in the past seven days and to rate the frequency of each item on a four-point scale: *never* (0), *rarely* (1), *sometimes* (2), and *often* (3). Items concerning negative thoughts, feelings and bodily experiences are reverse-scored so that when all 12 items are summed respondents can potentially score between 0 and 36, with higher scores indicating greater positive functioning. The PFI-12 is short and easy to complete.

The PFI-12 used the language of traditional psychology and psychiatry insofar as lower scores on the scale indicate greater problems of depression and anxiety, but instead of viewing these as categorical disorders, it presented these as

Table 9.1 Positive Functioning Inventory-12 (PFI-12)

A number of statements that people have made to describe how they feel are given below. Please read each one and tick the column which best describes how frequently you felt that way in the past seven days, including today. Some statements describe positive feelings and some describe negative feelings. You may have experienced both positive and negative feelings at different times during the past seven days.

		Never	Rarely	Sometimes	Often
1	I felt dissatisfied with my life.				
2	I felt happy.				
3	I felt cheerless.				
4	I felt pleased with the way I am.				
5	I felt that life was enjoyable.				
6	I felt that life was meaningless.				
7	I felt content.				
8	I felt tense.				
9	I felt calm.				
10	I felt relaxed.				
11	I felt upset.				
12	I felt worried.				

Scoring key: Items are scored as follows: never = 0, rarely = 1, sometimes = 2, often = 3.

Items 1, 3, 6, 8, 11 and 12 are reverse scored. Items 1 to 12 can be summed to provide a score for total positive functioning score.

problems in living, continuous with normal functioning, extending the idea of a continuum into the range of positive functioning, such that higher scores on the scale indicate greater well-being. As such the advantage of the PFI-12 over traditional self-report measures of depression and anxiety is that it not only allows us to assess the alleviation of depressive and anxious states, but also allows us to track the extent to which the client is moving towards positive functioning. For therapists who traditionally use measures of depression and anxiety but who have an interest in positive psychology the use of the PFI-12 may be useful.

The PFI-12 will be useful to practitioners and researchers who are in need of a short but reliable and valid measure of well-being. The PFI-12 provides clinicians with a rapid method of assessment with which to assess therapeutic change. There are now suggestions for various positive psychology interventions with clinical and health-related populations, and the PFI-12 promises to provide a useful tool for researchers wishing to assess the effectiveness of their interventions.

Scores on the PFI-12 can provide a useful summary of a client's progress. As with all such tools, clinical judgement is always important. Items are asked for in relation to their frequency. One might expect that most people who are functioning well in their lives will score relatively highly on the tool indicating that for most of the week they experienced more positive states than negative states. However, clinicians must always be cautious in how they interpret the scores of those who consistently score at the maximum. One cannot rule out the possibility that such a scoring pattern may in fact reflect an illusory or self-deceptive state in some. It is important in the interpretation of scores to take into account the context of a person's life and what affective, cognitive and bodily states are likely to be adaptive given their unique circumstances.

Unconditional positive self-regard

In contrast to positive psychology measures such as the one described above which build on the language of business-as-usual psychology to offer a new way of thinking, there are concepts in humanistic psychology that are already offering a positive psychological view. One such concept that, as we have already seen, is thought to be fundamental to the success of person-centred therapy is *unconditional positive self-regard* (UPSR).

UPSR refers to the individual's acceptance of all of his or her subjective experiences, without reference to either the perceived attitudes of others or to rules or values that have been internalized from the social environment. It involves relating to all of one's experiences, whether positive or negative, with warmth and a non-judgemental understanding. People differ in the extent to which they unconditionally regard themselves. A tool to help clinicians and researchers is the Unconditional Positive Self-Regard Scale (UPSRS: Patterson & Joseph 2006, 2013) (see Table 9.2).

The UPSR scale consists of twelve items. Six items refer to self-regard and six to conditionality. Responses to each item are rated on a five-point Likert-type scale ranging from 'strongly agree' to 'strongly disagree' and after taking reverse-scored items into account, a total score for each subscale is calculated. When scoring the UPSR scale, total scores are computed for each subscale but are not summated into a full-scale score, thus providing information about the two identified dimensions of unconditionality and positive self-regard.

Authenticity

One idea that is already central to humanistic and existential psychology that promises to be a cornerstone of the new positive clinical psychology is authenticity. Specifically, the Authenticity Scale (AS: Wood et al., 2008) was partially designed to be an outcome measure in therapy and a research tool consistent with person-centred psychology (Rogers, 1959). The AS is a positive psychological measure based on contemporary person-centred theory in which psychopathology, rather than being conceptualized from the perspective of psychiatric terminology, is viewed as arising through a lack of congruence between conscious awareness, inner emotional and cognitive states, and the social environment (Joseph & Worsley, 2005b).

Authenticity is conceptualized with a Tripartite Model, involving three components; (1) self-alienation, representing an inconsistent identity and the extent to which a person's self is incongruent with actual experiences and deeply held

Table 9.2 Unconditional Positive Self-Regard Scale (UPSR Scale)

Below is a list of statements dealing with your general feelings about yourself. Please respond to each statement by circling your answer using the scale '1 = Strongly disagree' to '5 = Strongly agree'.

	Strongly disagree	Disagree	Unsure	Agree	Strongly agree
1 I truly like myself.	1	2	3	4	5
2 Whether other people criticize me or praise me makes no real difference to the way I feel about myself.	1	2	3	4	5
3 There are certain things I like about myself and there are other things I don't like.	1	2	3	4	5
4 I feel that I appreciate myself as a person.	1	2	3	4	5
5 Some things I do make me feel good about myself whereas other things I do cause me to be critical of myself.	1	2	3	4	5
6 How I feel towards myself is not dependent on how others feel towards me.	1	2	3	4	5
7 I have a lot of respect for myself.	1	2	3	4	5
8 I feel deep affection for myself.	1	2	3	4	5
9 I treat myself in a warm and friendly way.	1	2	3	4	5
10 I don't think that anything I say or do really changes the way I feel about myself.	1	2	3	4	5
11 I really value myself.	1	2	3	4	5
12 Whether other people are openly appreciative of me or openly critical of me, it does not really change how I feel about myself.	1	2	3	4	5

Scoring Key: Items 3 and 5 are reverse scored.
Items 1 + 4 + 7 + 8 + 9 +11 = Self-regard subscale.
Items 2 + 3 + 5 + 6 + 10 + 12 = Conditionality subscale.

Scores have a possible range of 6 to 30 on each of the two subscales. On the 'Self-regard' subscale, high scores indicate presence of positive self-regard while low scores indicate absence of positive self-regard. On the 'Conditionality' subscale, high scores indicate *unconditionality* of self-regard, while low scores indicate *conditionality* of self-regard.

Table 9.3 Authenticity Scale

Please read the following statements and rate how well each describes you, where 1 = 'Does not describe me at all' and 7 = 'Describes me very well'.

_____ 1 I think it is better to be yourself, than to be popular.

_____ 2 I don't know how I really feel inside.

_____ 3 I am strongly influenced by the opinions of others.

_____ 4 I usually do what other people tell me to do.

_____ 5 I always feel I need to do what others expect me to do.

_____ 6 Other people influence me greatly.

_____ 7 I feel as if I don't know myself very well.

_____ 8 I always stand by what I believe in.

_____ 9 I am true to myself in most situations.

_____10 I feel out of touch with the 'real me'.

_____11 I live according to my values and beliefs.

_____12 I feel alienated from myself.

Scoring key: total items 3, 4, 5, 6 for external influences; 2, 7, 10 and 12 for self-alienation; and items 1, 8, 9 and 11 for authentic behaviour.

beliefs; (2) accepting external influence, instead of self-directing; and (3) authentic living, or behaving in ways consistent with beliefs and values (self-alienation and accepting external influence represent inauthenticity, whereas authentic living represents authenticity). Table 9.3 shows the Authenticity Scale.

The AS consists of twelve items which can be grouped into three subscales measuring resistance to external influence, self-alienation and authentic behaviour. Each item is rated in a seven-point scale such that scores on each subscale have a possible range of 4 to 28, with higher scores indicating greater external influence, greater self-alienation and greater authentic behaviour.

Growth following adversity

As we have seen in the previous chapter, post-traumatic growth has become a flagship topic for positive clinical psychology and is an idea that can be applied to a wide variety of life events.

The Psychological Well-Being–Post-Traumatic Changes Questionnaire (PWB–PTCQ: Joseph, Maltby, Wood, Stockton, Hunt, & Regel, 2012) was developed to assess post-traumatic growth (see Table 9.4).

Table 9.4 Psychological Well-Being–Post-Traumatic Change Questionnaire (PWB–PTCQ)

Think about how you feel about yourself at the present time. Please read each of the following statements and rate how you have changed as a result of the trauma.

5 = Much more so now
4 = A bit more so now
3 = I feel the same about this as before
2 = A bit less so now
1 = Much less so now

____ 1. I like myself.
____ 2. I have confidence in my opinions.
____ 3. I have a sense of purpose in life.
____ 4. I have strong and close relationships in my life.
____ 5. I feel I am in control of my life.
____ 6. I am open to new experiences that challenge me.
____ 7. I accept who I am, with both my strengths and limitations.
____ 8. I don't worry what other people think of me.
____ 9. My life has meaning.
____10. I am a compassionate and giving person.
____11. I handle my responsibilities in life well.
____12. I am always seeking to learn about myself.
____13. I respect myself.
____14. I know what is important to me and will stand my ground, even if others disagree.
____15. I feel that my life is worthwhile and that I play a valuable role in things.
____16. I am grateful to have people in my life who care for me.
____17. I am able to cope with what life throws at me.
____18. I am hopeful about my future and look forward to new possibilities.

Scoring key: Total all 18 statements.
Subscales: Self-acceptance (statements 1, 7 and 13), autonomy (statements 2, 8 and 14), purpose in life (statements 3, 9 and 15), relationships (statements 4, 10 and 16), sense of mastery (statements 5, 11 and 17), and personal growth (statements 6, 12 and 18).

The PWB–PTCQ consists of eighteen items. Respondents are asked to rate each on a five-point scale indicating to what extent they perceive themselves to have changed. Higher scores indicate greater positive changes. The highest score possible is 90. The lowest possible score is 18. Low scores indicate that the respondent perceives themselves to have diminished in psychological well-being. It is also possible to score the PWB–PTCQ according to the six domains of self-acceptance, autonomy, purpose in life, relationships, sense of mastery and openness to personal growth.

Research has shown that the PWB–PTCQ provides incremental validity over and above existing measures of growth following adversity in predicting levels of subjective well-being, has convergent validity with the newer positive psychology constructs of gratitude and authenticity, is not associated with social desirability and has a moderately strong correlation with actual changes in psychological well-being. The advantages of the PWB–PTCQ are that it provides a conceptual structure within which researchers and clinicians can integrate post-traumatic growth within the wider literature on well-being and positive psychology and it allows for respondents to rate how they have changed both positive and negative directions.

Challenges of measurement

Each of these tools offers a conceptualization of well-being which accommodates an understanding of distress and dysfunction and as such can be used as research and clinical outcome tools. For those who already routinely use measures in their practice the positive psychology agenda for measurement may be welcome. For other therapists the use of measures has traditionally been controversial because of their association with psychiatric diagnosis. As such there are a number of challenges that demand consideration.

Some in the person-centred community object to the use of measures, seeing their use as conflated with assessment and diagnosis (see Wilkins, 2005b). To the extent that measures are used to 'diagnose' and 'categorise' people, labelling them as suffering from this or that disorder, I would agree. Given that person-centred theory holds that psychopathology develops as a result of internalized conditions of worth and that amelioration of psychopathology takes place when the right social-environmental conditions are present, the approach to therapy remains the same regardless of what problem the person presents with. As such there is no need for diagnosis, which is only necessary within the medical model, which holds that psychological problems like medical problems require specific diagnosis in order to determine the appropriate specific treatment.

Person-centred therapists hold that diagnosis, formulation and assessment are unnecessary for the purpose of determining a course of therapy, as what is required will unfold in the here and now of the sessions. That is not to say that all person-centred therapists have exactly the same view. There will be different nuances in individuals' views on the use of diagnosis and assessment, depending on their work context, or other circumstances (see Wilkins, 2005b). But, on the whole, person-centred therapists do not routinely take case histories, assess, or diagnose their clients, as they do not make the assumption that there are specific treatments for specific problems. The therapist endeavours to offer an empathic, congruent and unconditionally accepting relationship across all clients.

Consequently, therapists may object to administering tests in the sense that this is a detraction from holding the above attitudinal conditions and from following the client's direction, and in this way I would agree that measurement is not a person-centred activity, per se. But I would also argue that there will be situations in which using such tools can be consistent with the client's direction. Person-centred therapy is an approach to therapy that says that the direction of therapy arises from the client and it is through the therapist's empathic understanding that the therapist is able to offer appropriate support for the direction of the client. I would argue that in the therapeutic relationship it may be appropriate at times to offer support for the client's autonomy development through the use of measures. If a client expresses an interest in learning about themselves in such a way that might be facilitated by the use of self-report questionnaires, and it is clear that this interest is coming from the client rather than me, then I will readily suggest to the client that it might be helpful to look at this or that exercise or measurement tool to assess their character strengths, or to give information on a topic.

So long as my agenda is about staying with the client and going in their direction this seems completely in accord with person-centred theory. What is important is that tests or other techniques are used as an expression of the necessary and sufficient conditions (Rogers, 1957) that constitute the therapeutic relationship. Some of the issues that clients bring to therapy lend themselves more to this than others. For many clients the conversation between us never develops in such a way that I would feel that it is anything but an interruption or distraction to the client's own direction to offer measures as a therapeutic vehicle. But with others I would be ignoring their direction if I did not offer something of myself or my knowledge in relation to their expressions of need, particularly so if they directly request such information from me.

In changing the outcomes that we are interested in, we also change the parameters of therapeutic engagement. Typically, clients perceive therapy as a time to talk about their distress and dysfunction and seek ways to find relief. But in changing the discourse to be about positive functioning or authenticity, for example, their expectations for therapy may change to include now explicitly seeking such positive changes. As such, not only are such measures of positive functioning useful in tracking change but they can also play a valuable therapeutic role if used skilfully and in the client's interests.

The use of assessment in this way is underpinned by two important caveats. First, it is always the case that assessment is offered to the client as a suggestion that can be taken up or not, rather than prescribed by the therapist as expert. This is crucial, since it underpins the fundamental principle of the person-centred approach to always be working to the client's agenda. Second, personality and strengths assessments are used in a facilitative way; they are not diagnostic. They open up areas for conversation and discussion, and can be swift and effective routes into those discussions. They are not used as ways of 'diagnosing', 'categorising', 'labelling', or otherwise imposing an external view on the person. Person-centred therapy was developed to facilitate people becoming more fully functioning. Many of the tests that are currently used are derived from other theoretical perspectives, and as such it is understandable that they are often seen as unhelpful. However, measurement does not imply diagnosis and it is theoretically compatible to ask clients about their levels of becoming fully functioning.

There are also strong practical reasons for the use of measures. Organizations demand evidence for the effectiveness of therapy. Within the structures of organizations in which measures are routinely administered in order to collect data to demonstrate the effects of the services provided to clients, there is little choice but to administer measures. Given that, the preference should be to use measures that are theoretically consistent with the nature of the therapy. In this respect person-centred therapists have a wealth of measures available from positive psychology that can be used to show the development of their clients towards becoming more fully functioning.By taking a creative and proactive approach to outcome measurement, person-centred therapists could identify and introduce theoretically and ethically consistent ways of demonstrating the effectiveness of therapy. This is exciting for the person-centred therapist who now has tools such as those mentioned above with which to assess change in the way that person-centred theory predicts.

Conclusion

While psychology has largely adopted psychiatric terminology, it is now important that practitioners begin to introduce positive functioning into their practice. In this chapter I have presented four scales which illustrate the different ways in which positive therapists can engage with this new agenda by using measures which are based on alternative conceptualizations of functioning. It is becoming ever more important to build evidence for positive change over the course of therapy. It is reasonable to expect that funders should want to see evidence for effectiveness. But how effectiveness is defined is not straightforward. Traditionally, it has been done using psychiatric terminology which has suited some forms of clinical practice but not all. However, we can now expect to see the way in which outcomes are defined change to include newer constructs drawn from positive psychology.

In this chapter, I have discussed how the use of tests and measures is controversial in the context of person-centred therapy when they are used from the perspective of the medical model. In person-centred therapy there is no need to diagnosis or assess from the perspective of the medical model as it is thought that, no matter what the presenting condition, it is the therapeutic relationship which is healing in all cases. Tests and measures derived from the positive psychology perspective can be useful in the context of therapy in helping the client's own self-understanding. But what is important is that the use of tests and measures are used from the client's frame of reference so that they remain their own best expert.

In the next chapter, my aim is to paint the canvas much more broadly, and go on to consider the social and political implications of the positive therapy approach, as well as addressing some of the issues of the sociocultural context of our work, and the need to be openly reflective about our therapeutic and professional practice.

Further reading

Patterson, T.G., & Joseph, S. (2007b). Outcome measurement in person-centered practice. In R. Worsley and S. Joseph (Eds) *Person-centered practice: Case studies in positive psychology* (pp. 200–217). Ross-on-Wye: PCCS Books.
The first chapter to explicitly argue for the use of theoretically consistent measures as a way for person-centred therapists to engage with the research agenda.

Joseph, S., & Wood, A. (2010). Assessment of positive functioning in clinical psychology: Theoretical and practical issues. *Clinical Psychology Review, 30*, 830–838.
A detailed discussion of the ways in which practitioners can engage with the agenda of positive psychology assessment.

Rashid, T. (2015). Strengths-based assessment. In S. Joseph (Ed.), *Positive psychology in practice: Promoting human flourishing in work, health, education, and everyday life* (2nd ed.) (pp. 519–542). Hoboken, NJ: Wiley.

Wood, A. M., Linley, P. A., Maltby, J., Baliousis, M., & Joseph, S. (2008). The authentic personality: A theoretical and empirical conceptualization and the development of the authenticity scale. *Journal of Counselling Psychology, 55*, 385–399.
An important paper because it develops a new positive psychology measure of authenticity based on person-centred theory, thus being one of the first papers to truly integrate the two disciplines.

Chapter 10

Conclusion

Reflections, challenges and the future

The first aim of this book was to show the relevance of positive psychology to therapy such that therapy no longer restricts itself to the alleviation of suffering, especially as defined by psychiatric categories, but sees its purpose as the facilitation of well-being, human flourishing and optimal functioning. The second was to show that person-centred therapy is an original positive psychology because of its focus on promoting fully functioning behaviour. The third was to show how person-centred theory and therapy is underpinned by the research and philosophy of self-determination theory (SDT) and other mainstream social and developmental psychology research. The fourth was to show how person-centred theory provides an integrative view of positive and negative experiences, in such a way to reconceptualize psychopathology as the thwarting of the human tendency towards flourishing. Finally, I wanted to make the case for the use of theory-consistent measures in research and practice instead of and alongside the traditional measures derived from the psychiatric model. I hope that I have achieved these aims. There are four challenges that arise that I will now discuss.

One

If you are a person-centred therapist I hope that you will have found what I have said encouraging and helpful. I think the general ideas of positive psychology to be concerned with optimal functioning resonate well with the person-centred approach and its research bolsters the evidence base for the person-centred approach.

The first challenge is for the person-centred community to realize they are part of positive psychology. Unless the person-centred community is open to engaging with the wider field and contemporary research in positive psychology my view is that it will struggle to survive as a distinct area of application. The person-centred approach must adapt and evolve with the times.

Two

At the seventh European Conference on Positive Psychology I facilitated a symposium entitled 'The legacy of Carl Rogers'. It showed me that there is now interest among many in the positive psychology community in the person-centred approach. But whereas the person-centred approach is by definition a positive psychology, positive psychology is not necessarily person-centred. Positive psychology is a broad discipline, attracting scholars united in their interest in optimal functioning, but with different theoretical perspectives.

I hope that if you are a positive psychologist interested in therapy that you will have found the book helpful. In the first instance positive psychology raised questions about the fundamental assumptions to do with human nature in therapy. Therapy is never neutral in its view of human nature. At core, as we have seen, is the idea that all therapists operate on the basis of deep-seated personal world views, or fundamental assumptions, that they bring into the consulting room, and which influence their way of being with another person.

Looking at the choice of assumptive frameworks, I proposed a positive therapeutic approach based on person-centred psychology and its concept of the actualizing tendency as the motivational force for optimal human development. The idea that the psyche contains its own natural or inherent principles that promote growth, integration and the resolution of psychological inconsistencies and conflicts is not a new one, but it is a powerful idea that resonates with contemporary positive psychological principles and is supported by emerging theory and research.

The second challenge of this book is to set out for yourself what your own fundamental assumptions are about human nature and to be able to articulate how your practice is consistent with those assumptions.

Three

With reflection on the above challenge I am sure that some will choose to reject the person-centred approach as not for them, but I hope that others will come to value and understand the person-centred approach and particularly the notion of non-directivity as the vehicle for self-determination. In part it is an intellectual challenge, but in other part it demands understanding from the inside out. The essence of and what defines person-centred therapy is the underlying assumption that distress and dysfunction arise when clients' inherent capacities for growth, fulfilment and well-being are thwarted by psychological and sociocultural factors. As such there is a belief in the self-determination of the client and that clients have the right answers for themselves. Therefore, forms of therapy which are prescriptive and structured in advance of meeting any particular client must by definition undermine their self-determination.

The logical position is for the therapist to be non-directive (Levitt, 2005b). As we have seen throughout this book, whether one chooses to adopt this approach comes down in the end to personal beliefs and fundamental assumptions about human nature. As Schmid (2005) wrote:

> Non-directivity is thus a matter of basic beliefs. People who think that direc-
> tivity is necessary in therapy and counselling have a different image of the
> human being, a different concept of how to deal with knowledge and a differ-
> ent ethical stance from those who work with their clients on the basis of non-
> directiveness. Since it is of no use to argue over beliefs (they precede acting,
> thinking, and science), there is no way to say who, ultimately, is right. (p. 82)

Non-directivity refers to the ambition of the therapist not to take precedence over
the client in determining the direction of what takes place in therapy. Most importantly, and I cannot emphasize this strongly enough, non-directivity does not
mean there is no direction – it is the therapist that is non-directive because he or
she is following the client's directions. Remember, the assumption is that clients
have inherent capacities for growth, fulfilment and well-being. As much as clients
may appear lost, confused and directionless, and look to others for direction, they
have direction within them. When clients are in the right social environment they
will begin to move in ways that do not seem lost, confused or directionless. As
a therapist one can only ever test this out for oneself by fully embracing whole-
heartedly the theory and the practice. To approach person-centred practice with
anything less than full commitment to the underlying assumption and the logical
position of trusting the client to find their way is not person-centred practice.

A non-directive attitude does not preclude the therapist introducing experiences for the client as part of the therapeutic process. It is in this way that we can
begin to envisage the marriage between positive psychology and person-centred
therapy with attention to process direction and person-activity fit. Self-determination
is developed when the therapist is able to facilitate the client in listening more
attentively to their own inner voice, i.e. to learn how to evaluate their experiences
from an internal locus rather than an external locus, thus freeing them to move
forward in life in new and constructive ways fully aware of their choices.

The third challenge is to understand that therapy in the person-centred tradition
is not about techniques but about the set of attitudes you hold. It is about empathy
towards yourself and others, being congruent in the sense of understanding yourself
and being genuine in your relationships, not holding that others should do or be anything different from how they are but regarding them with warmth as human beings
struggling to do their best to actualize. The task of the person-centred therapist,
from the moment on waking in the morning to falling asleep at night, is to live these
conditions as their way of being in the world. It is not always easy but the attitudinal
conditions described by Rogers are the person-centred therapist's compass point.

Four

The elephant in the room is the moral vision of psychotherapy. As Christopher
(1996) wrote:

When, as counselors, we interact with clients or engage in research or theorizing, we will be adopting a stance. This stance will be a moral stance, presupposing a moral vision. Whether we admit it or not in our work with clients, we are engaging in conversation about the good. Ultimately, counseling is part of a cultural discussion about ethos and world view, about the good life and the good person, and about moral visions. (1996, p. 24)

Rogers (1978) talked of the *quiet revolution* to describe the political agenda of how personal transformation leads to social change. As people change towards becoming more fully functioning, become more aware of their choices in life, and choose to pursue a life dictated by their own values, they will, according to Rogers, move towards becoming more socially constructive in their behaviour, thus more active politically, more open to the suffering of others, and more willing to engage at the social and political level.

But we must always be wary and on guard for when we are faced with a conflict between personal transformation and social control. Therapy is sometimes criticized for being part of the problem rather than the solution to society's problems. If people's problems arise because of poverty, corruption, poor education, unequal social systems and so on, then therapy after the fact is simply not the answer, because it is the social systems that need to be changed rather than the clients' thinking. Getting depressed people whose lives are blighted by poor housing, illness, poverty and so on to do gratitude exercises, for example, while ignoring their very real circumstances would seem misguided.

As the existential therapist Rollo May described, 'psychotherapists become the agents of the culture whose particular task it is to adjust people to it: psychotherapy becomes an expression of the fragmentation of the period rather than an enterprise for overcoming it' (1958, p. 87). Therapy after the fact becomes part of the problem insofar as it is used to prop up existing and harmful social systems. The danger is that we deceive ourselves into believing that we are agents of personal transformation when we are in fact agents of social control (Murphy, Duggan, & Joseph, 2013a). In this respect, therapy is controversial. Much less so, in my view, are non-directive therapies that see the client as the best expert on their situation and do not decide in advance in what way the client needs to change.

This fourth challenge is for positive psychologists and person-centred therapists to consider their work within the wider cultural context and to be on the lookout for the inevitable tensions between the competing agendas of personal transformation and social control.

Conclusion

For me, the person-centred approach has provided a view of human nature which seems most in keeping with the world I see around me and a way of being that seems worth aspiring to morally. I view myself as a positive psychologist and as a person-centred therapist. As a positive psychologist I am influenced by the theoretical view of the person-centred approach that human beings are essentially constructive and motivated towards growth, and all the attendant implications for practice that go with this. As a person-centred therapist I am influenced by positive psychology to focus on fully functioning rather than treatment for psychiatric diagnosis with all its implications of science and measurement.

Finally, my argument in this book has been that it is not so much about 'what' the therapist does, but rather it is about 'how' they do it, or more accurately, 'how the therapist is being in relationship with the client', that is important. Therapists who value and accept their clients as agents of self-determination and are able to relate to them at depth are doing what I would call positive therapy.

Useful websites

World Association for Person-Centered & Experiential Psychotherapy & Counseling.
http://www.pce-world.org/

European Network for Positive Psychology.
http://www.enpp.eu/

International Positive Psychology Association.
http://www.ippanetwork.org/

The British Association for the Person-Centred Approach.
http://www.bapca.org.uk/

References

Abraido-Lanza, A. F., Guier, C., & Colon, R. M. (1998). Psychological thriving among Latinas with chronic illness. *Journal of Social Issues, 54*, 405–424.

Ackerman, S. J., & Hilsenroth, M. J. (2003). A review of therapist characteristics and techniques positively impacting the therapeutic alliance. *Clinical Psychology Review, 23*, 1–33.

Adler, A. (1927). *The practice and theory of individual psychology.* New York: Harcourt, Brace & World.

Affleck, G., & Tennen, H. (1996). Construing benefits from adversity: Adaptational significance and dispositional underpinnings. *Journal of Personality, 64*, 899–922.

Albee, G. W. (2000). The Boulder model's fatal flaw. *American Psychologist, 55*, 247–248.

Aldwin, C. M. (1994). Transformational coping. In C. M. Aldwin (Ed.), *Stress, coping, and development* (pp. 240–269). New York: Guilford.

American Psychiatric Association. (2013). *Diagnostic and statistical manual of mental disorders* (5th ed.). Washington, DC: American Psychiatric Press.

American Psychological Association. (2013). *Society of counseling psychology: President's welcome.* http://www.div17.org/about/presidents-welcome, accessed on 14.09.2013.

Andrews, F. M., & Withey, S. B. (1976). *Social indicators of well-being: America's perception of life quality.* New York: Plenum.

Angyal, A. (1941). *Foundations for a science of personality.* New York: Commonwealth Fund.

Antonovsky, A. (1987). *Unravelling the mystery of health: How people manage stress and stay well.* San Francisco: Jossey-Bass.

Armeli, S., Gunthert, K. C., & Cohen, L. H. (2001). Stressor appraisals, coping, and post-event outcomes: The dimensionality and antecedents of stress-related growth. *Journal of Social and Clinical Psychology, 20*, 366–395.

Aspinwall, L. G., & Staudinger, U. M. (Eds). (2003). *A psychology of human strengths: Fundamental questions and future directions for a positive psychology.* Washington, DC: American Psychological Association.

Assor, A., Roth, G., & Deci, E. L. (2004). The emotional costs of parents' conditional regard: A self-determination theory analysis. *Journal of Personality, 72*, 47–88.

Baer, R. (2003). Mindfulness training as a clinical intervention: A conceptual and empirical review. *Clinical Psychology: Science and Practice, 10*, 125–143.

Baker, N. (2004). Experiential person-centred therapy. In P. Sanders, *The tribes of the person-centred nation: An introduction to the schools of therapy related to the person-centred approach* (pp. 67–94). Ross-on-Wye: PCCS Books:

Barret-Kruse, C. (1994). Brief counselling: A user's guide for traditionally trained counsellors. *International Journal for the Advancement of Counselling, 17*, 109–115.

Barrett-Lennard, G. T. (1986). The relationship inventory now: Issues and advances in theory, method and use. In L. S. Greenberg & W. M. Pinsof (Eds), *The psychotherapeutic process: A research handbook* (pp. 439–476). New York: Guilford Press.

Barrett-Lennard, G. T. (1998). *Carl Rogers' helping system: Journey and substance.* London: Sage.

Bishop, S. R., Lau, M., Shapiro, S., Carlson, L., Anderson, N. D., Carmody, J., & Devins, G. (2004). Mindfulness: A proposed operational definition. *Clinical Psychology: Science and Practice, 11*, 230–241.

Bohart, A. C. (2013). The actualising person. In M. Cooper, P. F. Schmid, M. O'Hara, & A. C. Bohart (Eds), *The handbook of person-centred psychotherapy and counselling* (2nd ed.) (pp. 84–101). Basingstoke: Palgrave.

Bohart, A. C., O'Hara, M., & Leitner, L. M. (1998). Empirically violated treatments: Disenfranchisement of humanistic and other psychotherapies. *Psychotherapy Research, 8*, 141–157.

Bolt, M. (2004). *Pursuing human strengths: A positive psychology guide.* New York: Worth.

Boniwell, I., Kauffman, C., & Silberman, J. (2014). The positive psychology approach to coaching. In E. Cox, T. Bachkirova, & D. Clutterbuck (Eds), *The complete handbook of coaching* (2nd ed.) (pp. 157–169). London: Sage.

Bozarth, J. D., & Motomasa, N. (2005). Searching for the core: The interface of client-centered principles with other therapies. In S. Joseph & R. Worsley (Eds), *Person-centred psychopathology: A positive psychology of mental health.* Ross-on-Wye: PCCS books.

Bozarth, J. D. (1998). *Person-centred therapy: A revolutionary paradigm.* Ross-on-Wye: PCCS Books.

Bozarth, J. D., & Wilkins, P. (Eds). (2001). *Unconditional positive regard: Rogers' therapeutic conditions: Evolution, theory and practice. Vol. 3.* Ross-on-Wye: PCCS Books.

Brazier, D. (1993). Introduction. In D. Brazier (Ed.), *Beyond Carl Rogers: Towards a psychotherapy for the 21st century.* London: Constable.

Brazier, D. (1995). *Zen therapy.* London: Constable.

Bretherton, R. (2015). Existential dimensions of positive psychology. In S. Joseph (Ed.), *Positive psychology in practice: Promoting human flourishing in work, health, education and everyday life* (2nd ed.) (pp. 47–59). Hoboken, NJ: Wiley.

Bretherton, R., & Ørner, R. (2003). Positive psychotherapy in disguise. *The Psychologist, 16*, 136–137.

Bretherton, R., & Ørner, R. J. (2004). Positive psychology and psychotherapy: An existential approach. In P. A. Linley & S. Joseph (Eds), *Positive psychology in practice* (pp. 420–430). Hoboken: Wiley.

Brodley, B. T. (2005a). Client-centered values limit the application of research findings: An issue for discussion. In S. Joseph & R. Worsley (Eds), *Person-centred psychopathology: A positive psychology of mental health* (pp. 310–316). Ross-on-Wye: PCCS books.

Brodley, B. T. (2005b). About the non-directive attitude. In B. E. Levitt (Ed.), *Embracing non-directivity: Reassessing person-centered theory and practice in the 21st century* (pp. 1–4). Ross-on-Wye: PCCS books.

Brown, K. W., & Ryan, R. M. (2003). The benefits of being present: Mindfulness and its role in psychological well-being. *Journal of Personality and Social Psychology, 84*, 822–848.

Brown, K. W., & Ryan, R. M. (2004). Fostering healthy self-regulation from within and without: A self-determination theory perspective. In P. A. Linley & S. Joseph (Eds), *Positive psychology in practice* (pp. 105–124). Hoboken: Wiley.

Calhoun, L. G., Cann, A., Tedeschi, R. G., & McMillan, J. (2000). A correlational test of the relationship between posttraumatic growth, religion, and cognitive processing. *Journal of Traumatic Stress, 13*, 521–527.

Calhoun, L. G., & Tedeschi, R. G. (1999). *Facilitating posttraumatic growth: A clinician's guide.* Mahwah, NJ: Lawrence Erlbaum.

Cameron, K. S., Dutton, J. E., & Quinn, R. E. (Eds). (2003). *Positive organizational scholarship: Foundations of a new discipline.* San Francisco, CA: Berrett-Koehler.

Carr, A. (2003). *Positive psychology: The science of happiness and human strengths.* London: Brunner-Routledge.

Carver, C. S., & Baird, E. (1998). The American dream revisited: Is it *what* you want or *why* you want it that matters? *Psychological Science, 9*, 289–292.

Chan, R., & Joseph, S. (2000). Dimensions of personality, domains of aspiration, and subjective well-being. *Personality and individual differences, 28*, 347–354.

Chirkov, V., Ryan, R. M., Kim, Y., & Kaplan, U. (2003). Differentiating autonomy from individualism and independence: A self-determination perspective on internalization of cultural orientations, gender, and well-being. *Journal of Personality and Social Psychology, 84*, 97–110.

Chouliara, Z., Karatzias, T., Scott-Brien, G., Macdonald, A., MacArthur, & Frazer, N. (2012). Adult survivors' of childhood sexual abuse perspectives of services: A systematic review. *Counselling and Psychotherapy Research: Linking research with practice, 12*, 146–161.

Christopher, J. C. (1996). Counseling's inescapable moral visions. *Journal of Counseling and Development, 75*, 17–25.

Christopher, M. (2004). A broader view of trauma: A biopsychosocial-evolutionary view of the role of the traumatic stress response in the emergence of pathology and/or growth. *Clinical Psychology Review, 24*, 75–98.

Compton, W. C. (2004). *An introduction to positive psychology.* Belmont, CA: Wadsworth.

Compton, W. C., Smith, M. L., Cornish, K. A., & Qualls, D. L. (1996). Factor structure of mental health measures. *Journal of Personality and Social Psychology, 71*, 406–413.

Cooper, M., Joseph, S. (in press). Psychological foundations for humanistic psychotherapeutic practice. In D. A. Cain, K. Keenan, & S. Rubin (Eds). *Handbook of humanistic psychotherapies.* Washington, DC: American Psychological Association.

Cooper, M., O'Hara, M., Schmid, P. F., & Bohart, A. C. (Eds). (2013). *The handbook of person-centred psychotherapy and counselling* (2nd ed.). Basingstoke: Palgrave

Corcoran, K., & Fischer, J. (2000). *Measures for clinical practice* (2nd ed.). New York: The Free Press.

Cornelius-White, J. H. D. (2002). The phoenix of empirically supported therapy relationships: The overlooked person-centered basis. *Psychotherapy: Theory/research/practice/training, 39*, 219–222.

Creamer, M., Burgess, P., & Pattison, P. (1992). Reaction to trauma: A cognitive processing model. *Journal of Abnormal Psychology, 101*, 452–459.

Crocker, J., Luhtanen, R. K., Cooper, M. L., & Bouvrette, A. (2003). Contingencies of self-worth in college students: Theory and measurement. *Journal of Personality and Social Psychology, 85*, 894–908.

Crocker, J., & Wolfe, C. T. (2001). Contingencies of self-worth. *Psychological Review, 108*, 593–623.

Csikszentmihalyi, M. (1990). *Flow: The psychology of optimal experience*. New York: Harper & Row.

Csikszentmihalyi, M. (1997). *Finding flow: The psychology of engagement with everyday life*. New York: Basic books.

Csikszentmihalyi, M. (1999). If we are so rich, why aren't we happy? *American Psychologist, 54*, 821–827.

Csikszentmihalyi, M. (2003). Legs or wings? A reply to R. S. Lazarus. *Psychological Inquiry, 14*, 113–115.

Csikszentmihalyi, M., & Rochberg-Halton, E. (1981). *The meaning of things. Domestic symbols and the self*. Cambridge, MA: Cambridge University Press.

Csikszentmihalyi, M., & Csikszentmihalyi, I. S. (Eds). (2006). *A life worth living: Contributions to positive psychology*. New York: Oxford University Press.

Csillik, A. S. (2013). Understanding motivational interviewing effectiveness: Contributions from Rogers' client-centered approach. *Journal of Humanistic Psychology, 41*, 350–363.

David, S. A., Boniwell, I., & Conley Ayers, A. (Eds). (2013). *The Oxford handbook of happiness*. Oxford: Oxford University Press.

Davis, C. G., Nolen-Hoeksema, S., & Larson, J. (1998). Making sense of loss and benefiting from the experience: Two construals of meaning. *Journal of Personality and Social Psychology, 75*, 561–574.

Deci, E. L., Koestner, R., & Ryan, R. M. (1999). A meta-analytic review of experiments examining the effects of extrinsic rewards on intrinsic motivation. *Psychological Bulletin, 25*, 627–668.

Deci, E. L., & Ryan, R. M. (1985). *Intrinsic motivation and self-determination in human behavior*. New York: Plenum.

Deci, E. L., & Ryan, R. M. (1991). A motivational approach to self: Integration in personality. In R. Dienstbier (Ed.), *Nebraska symposium on motivation, Vol. 38. Perspectives on motivation* (pp. 237–288). Lincoln, NE: University of Nebraska Press.

Deci, E. L., & Ryan, R. M., (1995). Human Agency: The basis for true self-esteem. In M.H.Kernis (Ed.), *Efficacy, agency, and self-esteem* (pp. 31–50). New York: Plenum.

Deci, E. L., & Ryan, R. M. (2000). The 'what' and 'why' of goal pursuits: Human needs and the self-determination of behavior. *Psychological Inquiry, 4*, 227–268.

Deci, E. L., & Vansteenkiste, M. (2004). Self-determination theory and basic need satisfaction: Understanding human development in positive psychology. *Ricerche di psicologia: Special issue in positive psychology, 27*, 23–40.

Delle Fave, A., & Massimini, F. (2004). Bringing subjectivity into focus: Optimal experiences, life themes, and person-centered rehabilitation. In P. A. Linley & S.Joseph (Eds), *Positive psychology in practice* (pp. 581–597). Hoboken, NJ: Wiley.

Department of Health (2000). *The NHS cancer plan*. London: Department of Health.

Deurzen, E. (1998). Beyond psychotherapy. *Psychotherapy section newsletter of the British Psychological Society, 23*, 4–18.

Diener, E., & Seligman, M. E. P. (2004). Beyond money: Toward an economy of well-being. *Psychological Science in the Public Interest, 5*, 1–31.

Donlevy, J. G. (1996). Jung's contribution to adult development: The difficult and misunderstood path of individuation. *Journal of Humanistic Psychology, 36*, 92–108.

Duncan, B., & Miller, S. (2000). *The heroic client: Doing client-directed, outcome informed therapy*. San Francisco, CA: Jossey-Bass.

Elliott, R., Greenberg, L. S., Watson, J., Timulak, L., & Freire, B. (2013). Research on humanistic-experiential psychotherapies. In M. J. Lambert (Ed.), *Bergin & S.L. Garfield's handbook of psychotherapy and behavior change* (6th ed.). New York: Wiley & Sons.

Farber, B. A., Brink, D. C., & Raskin, P. M. (Eds). (1996). *The psychotherapy of Carl Rogers: Cases and commentary*. New York: Guilford.

Fava, G. A. (1997). Conceptual obstacles to research progress in affective disorders. *Psychotherapy and Psychosomatics, 66*, 283–285.

Fava, G. A. (1999). Well-being therapy. *Psychotherapy and Psychosomatics, 68*, 171–178.

Fava, G. A. (2000). Cognitive behavioral therapy. In M. Fink (Ed.), *Encyclopedia of stress* (pp. 484–497). San Diego, CA: Academic Press.

Fava, G. A., Rafanelli, C., Cazzaro, M., Conti, S., & Grandi, S. (1998). Well-being therapy: A novel psychotherapeutic approach for residual symptoms of affective disorders. *Psychological Medicine, 28*, 475–480.

Fava, G. A., Rafanelli, C., Grandi, S., Conti, S., & Belluardo, P. (1998). Prevention of recurrent depression with cognitive-behavioral therapy. *Archives of General Psychiatry, 55*, 816–820.

Fava, G. A., Ruini, C., Rafanelli, C., Finos, L., Salmaso, L., Mangelli, L., & Sirigatti, S. (2005). Well-being therapy of generalized anxiety disorder. *Psychotherapy and Psychosomatics, 74*, 26–30.

Fava, G. A., Ruini, C., Rafanelli, C., & Grandi, S. (2002). Cognitive behavior approach to loss of clinical effect during long-term antidepressant treatment. *American Journal of Psychiatry, 159*, 2094–2095.

Foa, E. B., Keane, T. M., & Friedman, M. J. (Eds). (2000). *Effective treatments for PTSD: Practice guidelines from the International Society for Traumatic Stress Studies*. New York: Guilford Press.

Foa, E. B., & Kozak, M. J. (1986). Emotional processing of fear: Exposure to corrective information. *Psychological Bulletin, 99*, 20–35.

Foa, E. B., & Rothbaum, B. O. (1998). *Treating the trauma of rape: Cognitive-behavioral therapy for PTSD*. New York: Guilford.

Folkman, S., & Moskowitz, J. T. (2003). Positive psychology from a coping perspective. *Psychological Inquiry, 14*, 121–125.

Ford, J. G. (1991). Rogerian self-actualization: a clarification of meaning. *Journal of Humanistic Psychology, 31*, 101–111.

Frankl, V. (1963). *Man's search for meaning: An introduction to logotherapy*. New York: Pocket Books.

Fredrickson, B. L. (1998). What good are positive emotions? *Review of General Psychology, 2*, 300–319.

Fredrickson, B. L. (2001). The role of positive emotions in positive psychology: The broaden-and-build theory of positive emotions. *American Psychologist, 56*, 218–226.

Fredrickson, B. L., & Levenson, R. W. (1998). Positive emotions speed recovery from the cardiovascular sequelae of negative emotions. *Cognition and Emotion, 12*, 191–220.

Freire, E., Elliott, R., & Westwell, G. (2013). Person-centred and experiential psychotherapy scale: Development and reliability of an adherence/competence measure for person-centred and experiential psychotherapies. *Counselling and Psychotherapy Research*. DOI: 10.1080/14733145.2013.808682.

Fromm, E. (1976). *To have or to be*? New York: Harper & Row.

Gable, S. L., & Haidt, J. (2005). What (and why) is positive psychology? *Review of General Psychology, 9*, 103–110.

Gendlin, E. T. (1996) *Focusing-oriented psychotherapy: A manual of the experiential method*. New York: Guilford.

Geuter, U. (1992). *The professionalism of psychology in Nazi Germany*. Cambridge: Cambridge University Press.

Gilbert, P., & Irons, C. (2009). Compassion-focused therapies and compassionate mind training for shame and self attacking. In P. Gilbert (Ed.), *Compassion: Conceptualisations, research and use in psychotherapy* (pp. 263–325). London: Routledge

Goldstein, K. (1939). *The organism*. New York: American Books.

Grant, B. (1990). Principled and instrumental nondirectiveness in person-centred and client-centered therapy. *Person-Centered Review, 5* (1), 77–88. Reprinted in D. Cain (Ed.). (2002) *Classics in the person-centered approach* (pp. 371–377). Ross-on-Wye: PCCS Books.

Grant, B. (2004). The imperative of ethical justification in psychotherapy: The special case of client-centered therapy. *Person-Centered and Experiential Psychotherapies, 3*, 152–165.

Greenberg, L. S., Elliott, R., & Lietaer, G. (1994). Research on humanistic and experiential psychotherapies. In A. E. Bergin & S. L. Garfield (Eds), *Handbook of psychotherapy and behavior change* (4th ed.) (pp. 509–539). New York: Wiley.

Greenberg, L. S., Rice, L. N., & Elliott, R. (1993). *Facilitating emotional change: The moment by moment process*. New York: Guilford Press.

Grossman, P., Niemann, L., Schmidt, S., & Walach, H. (2004). Mindfulness-based stress reduction and health benefits. *Journal of Psychosomatic Medicine, 57*, 35–43.

Hansard, C. (2001). *The Tibetan art of living: Wise body, wise mind, wise life*. London: Hodder & Stoughton.

Harlow, H. F. (1953). Mice, monkeys, men, and motives. *Psychological Review, 60*, 23–32.

Harter, S., Marold, D. B., Whitesell, N. R., & Cobbs, G. (1996). A model of the effects of parent and peer support on adolescent false self behavior. *Child Development, 67*, 360–374.

Haugh, S., & Merry, T. (Eds). (2001). *Rogers' therapeutic conditions: Evolution, theory and practice. Vol. 2: Empathy*. PCCS Books: Ross-on-Wye.

Heelas, P., & Lock, A. (Eds). (1981). *Indigenous psychologies: The anthropology of the self*. New York: Academic.

Hefferon, K., & Boniwell, I. (2011). *Positive psychology: Theory, research and applications*. Maidenhead: Open University.

Held, B. S. (2002). The tyranny of the positive attitude in America: Observation and speculation. *Journal of Clinical Psychology, 58*, 965–992.

Herman, J. L. (1992). *Trauma and recovery: From domestic abuse to political terror*. London: Pandora.

Hodges, T. D., & Clifton, D. O. (2004). Strengths based development in practice. In P. A. Linley, & S. Joseph (Eds), *Positive psychology in practice* (pp. 256–268). Hoboken: Wiley.

Horney, K. (1951). *Neurosis and human growth: The struggle toward self-realization*. London: Routledge & Kegan Paul Ltd.

Horowitz, M. J. (1982). Psychological processes induced by illness, injury, and loss. In T. Millon, C. Green, & R. Meagher (Eds), *Handbook of clinical health psychology* (pp. 53–68). New York: Plenum.

Horowitz, M. J. (1986). *Stress response syndromes*. Northville, NJ: Jason Aronson.

Hubble, M. A., & Miller, S. D. (2004). The client: Psychotherapy's missing link for promoting a positive psychology. In P. A. Linley, & S. Joseph (Eds), *Positive psychology in practice* (pp. 335–353). Hoboken, NJ: Wiley.

Huppert, F. A. (2004). A population approach to positive psychology: The potential for population interventions to promote well-being and prevent disorder. In P. A. Linley, & S. Joseph (Eds), *Positive psychology in practice* (pp. 693–709). Hoboken, NJ: Wiley.

Huta, V. (2015). The complementary roles of eudaimonia and hedonia and how they can be pursued in practice. In S. Joseph (Ed.), *Positive Psychology in Practice: Promoting human flourishing in work, health, education and everyday life* (2nd ed.) (pp. 159–182). Hoboken, NJ: Wiley.

Huta, V., & Ryan, R. M. (2010). Pursuing pleasure or virtue: The differential and overlapping well-being benefits of hedonic and eudaimonic motives. *Journal of Happiness Studies, 11*, 735–762.

Huta, V., & Waterman A. S. (2014). Eudaimonia and its distinction from hedonia: Developing a classification and terminology for understanding conceptual and operational definitions. *Journal of Happiness Studies, 15* (6), 1425–1456.

Jaffe, D. T. (1985). Self-renewal: Personal transformation following extreme trauma. *Journal of Humanistic Psychology, 25*, 99–124.

James, W. (1902). *The varieties of religious experience: A study in human nature.* New York: Longman, Green.

Janoff-Bulman, R. (1989). Assumptive worlds and the stress of traumatic events: Applications of the schema construct. *Social Cognition, 7*, 113–136.

Janoff-Bulman, R. (1992). *Shattered assumptions: Towards a new psychology of trauma.* New York: Free Press.

Janoff-Bulman, R., & McPherson Frantz, C. (1997). The impact of trauma on meaning: From meaningless world to meaningful life. In M. Power & C. R. Brewin (Eds), *The transformation of meaning in psychological therapies.* Chichester: Wiley.

Joseph, S. (1999). Attributional processes, coping, and post-traumatic stress disorders. In W. Yule. (Ed.), *Post-traumatic stress disorders: Concepts and therapy* (pp. 51–70). Chichester: Wiley.

Joseph, S. (2003a). Client-centred psychotherapy: Why the client knows best. *The Psychologist, 16*, 304–307.

Joseph, S. (2003b). Person-centred approach to understanding posttraumatic stress. *Person-Centred Practice, 11*, 70–75.

Joseph, S. (2004). Client-centred therapy, post-traumatic stress, and post-traumatic growth: Theoretical perspectives and practical implications. *Psychology and Psychotherapy: Theory, Research and Practice, 77*, 101–120.

Joseph, S. (2005). Understanding post-traumatic stress from the person-centred perspective. In S. Joseph and R. Worsley (Eds), *Person-centred psychopathology: A positive psychology of mental health* (pp. 190–201). Ross-on-Wye: PCCS Books.

Joseph, S. (2006). Person-centred coaching psychology: A meta-theoretical perspective. *International Coaching Psychology Review, 1*, 47–55.

Joseph, S. (2010). *Theories of counselling and psychotherapy: An introduction.* Houndmills: Palgrave Macmillan.

Joseph, S. (2011). *What doesn't kill us: The new psychology of posttraumatic growth.* New York: Basic Books.

Joseph, S. (Ed.). (2015). *Positive psychology in practice: Promoting human flourishing in work, health, education and everyday life* (2nd ed.). Hoboken, NJ: Wiley.

Joseph, S., & Linley, P. A. (2004). Positive therapy: A positive psychological theory of therapeutic practice. In P. A. Linley & S. Joseph (Eds), *Positive psychology in practice* (pp. 354–368). Hoboken, NJ: Wiley.

Joseph, S., & Linley, P. A. (2005). Positive adjustment to threatening events: An organismic valuing theory of growth through adversity. *Review of General Psychology, 9*, 262–280.

Joseph, S., & Linley, P. A. (2008a), (Eds). *Trauma, recovery, and growth: Positive psychological perspectives on posttraumatic stress.* Hoboken, NJ: John Wiley & Sons.

Joseph, S. & Linley, P. A. (2008b). Psychological assessment of growth following adversity: A review. In S. Joseph, & P. A. Linley, (Eds). *Trauma, recovery, and growth: Positive psychological perspectives on posttraumatic stress* (pp. 21–38). Hoboken, NJ: John Wiley & Sons.

Joseph, S., Linley, P. A., Andrews, L., Harris, G., Howle, B., Woodward, C., & Shevlin, M. (2005). Assessing positive and negative changes in the aftermath of adversity: Psychometric evaluation of the Changes in Outlook Questionnaire. *Psychological Assessment, 17*, 70–80.

Joseph, S., Linley, P. A., Shevlin, M., Goodfellow, B., & Butler, L. (2006). Assessing positive and negative changes in the aftermath of adversity: A short form of the changes in Outlook Questionnaire. *Journal of loss and Trauma, 11*, 85–89.

Joseph, S., & Maltby, J. (2014). Positive functioning inventory: Initial validation of a 12-item self-report measure of well-being. *Psychology of Well-Being: Theory, Research and Practice, 4*, 15

Joseph, S., Maltby, J., Wood, A.M., Stockton, H., Hunt, N., & Regel, S. (2012). The psychological well-being–post traumatic changes questionnaire (PWB–PTCQ): Reliability and validity. *Psychological Trauma: Theory, Research, Practice, and Policy, 4*, 420–428

Joseph, S., & Murphy, D. (2013a). Person-centered theory encountering mainstream psychology: Building bridges and looking to the future. In J. H. D. Cornelius-White, R. Motschnig-Pitrik, & M. Lux (Eds), *Interdisciplinary handbook of the person-centered approach: Research and theory* (pp. 213–226). New York: Springer.

Joseph, S., & Murphy, D. (2013b). Person-centered approach, positive psychology and relational helping: Building bridges. *Journal of Humanistic Psychology, 53*, 26–51.

Joseph, S., Murphy, D., & Regel, S. (2012). An affective-cognitive processing model for post-traumatic growth. *Clinical Psychology and Psychotherapy, 19*, 316–325

Joseph, S., & Patterson, T. G. (2008). The actualising tendency: A meta-theoretical perspective for positive psychology. In B. E. Levitt (Ed.), *Reflections on human potential* (pp. 1–16). Ross-on Wye: PCCS Books.

Joseph, S., Williams, R., & Yule, W. (1993). Changes in outlook following disaster: The preliminary development of a measure to assess positive and negative responses. *Journal of Traumatic Stress, 6*, 271–279.

Joseph, S., Williams, R., & Yule, W. (1997). *Understanding post-traumatic stress: A psychosocial perspective on PTSD and treatment.* Chichester: Wiley.

Joseph, S., & Worsley, R. (Eds). (2005a). *Person-centred psychopathology: A positive psychology of mental health.* Ross-on-Wye: PCCS Books.

Joseph, S., & Worsley, R. (2005b). A positive psychology of mental health: The person-centred perspective. In S. Joseph & R. Worsley (Eds), *Person-centred psychopathology: A positive psychology of mental health* (pp. 348–357). Ross-on-Wye: PCCS Books.

Judge, T. A., Thoresen, C. J., Bono, J. E., & Patton, G. K. (2001). The job satisfaction-job performance relationship: A qualitative and quantitative review. *Psychological Bulletin, 127*, 376–407.

Jung, C. G. (1933). *Modern man in search of a soul.* New York: Harcourt, Brace, & World.

Kabat-Zinn, J. (1994). *Wherever you go, there you are.* New York, NY: Hyperion.

Kabat-Zinn, J. (2013). *Full catastophe living: Using the wisdom of your body and mind to face stress, pain and illness* (Rev. ed.). New York, NY: Bantam.

Kasser, T. (2002). *The high price of materialism.* Cambridge, MA: MIT Press.

Kasser, T. (2015). The science of values in the culture of consumption. In S. Joseph (Ed.), *Positive psychology in practice: Promoting human flourishing in work, health, education and everyday life* (2nd ed.) (pp. 83–102). Hoboken, NJ: Wiley.

Kasser, T., & Ryan, R. M. (1993). A dark side of the American dream: Correlates of financial success as a central life aspiration. *Journal of Personality and Social Psychology, 65*, 410–422.

Kasser, T., & Ryan, R. M. (1996). Further examining the American dream: Differential correlates of intrinsic and extrinsic goals. *Personality and Social Psychology Bulletin, 22*, 280–287.

Kasser, T., Ryan, R. M., Zax, M., & Sameroff, A. J. (1995). The relations of material and social environments to late adolescents' materialistic and prosocial values. *Developmental Psychology, 31*, 907–914.

Kauffman, C. (2005). You are just p.e.r.f.e.c.t. A positive psychology perspective of multiple resources. Paper presented at the American Psychological Association, Washington DC.

Kauffman, C., & Scoular, A. (2004). Toward a positive psychology of executive coaching. In P. A. Linley, & S. Joseph (Eds), *Positive psychology in practice* (pp. 287–302). Hoboken, NJ: Wiley.

Kearney, A. (1996). *Counselling, class and politics: Undeclared influences in therapy.* Ross-on-Wye: PCCS books.

Kekes, J. (1995). *Moral wisdom and good lives.* Ithaca, NY: Cornell University Press.

Kessler, B. G. (1987). Bereavement and personal growth. *Journal of Humanistic Psychology, 27*, 228–247.

Keyes, C. L. M., & Haidt, J. (Eds). (2002). *Flourishing: Positive psychology and the life well-lived.* Washington, DC: American Psychological Association.

Keyes, C. L. M., Shmotkin, D., & Ryff, C. D. (2002). Optimizing well-being: The empirical encounter of two traditions. *Journal of Personality and Social Psychology, 82*, 1007–1022.

Kidner, D. (2001). Silence is a political act: Letters to the editor. *The Psychologist, 14*, 178.

Kirschenbaum, H. (2007). *The life and work of Carl Rogers.* Ross-on-Wye: PCCS Books.

Koenig, H. G., Pargament, K. I., & Nielsen, J. (1998). Religious coping and health status in medically ill hospitalized older adults. *Journal of Nervous and Mental Disease, 186*, 513–521.

Korchin, S. J. (1976). *Modern clinical psychology.* New York: Basic Books.

La Guardia, J. G., Ryan, R. M., Couchman, C. E., & Deci, E. L. (2000). Within-person variation in security of attachment: A self-determination theory perspective on attachment, need fulfilment, and well-being. *Journal of Personality and Social Psychology, 79*, 367–384.

Lavender, T. (2003). Redressing the balance: The place, history and future of reflective practice in training. *Clinical Psychology, 27*, 11–15.

Layous, K., Sheldon, K. M., & Lyubomirsky, S. (2015). The prospects, practices, and prescriptions for the pursuit of happiness. In S. Joseph (Ed.), *Positive psychology in practice: Promoting human flourishing in work, health, education and everyday life.* (2nd ed.) (pp. 185–205). Hoboken, NJ: Wiley.

Lazarus, R. S. (2003). Does the positive psychology movement have legs? *Psychological Inquiry, 14*, 93–109.

Lazarus, R. S., & Folkman, S. (1984). *Stress, appraisal, and coping.* New York: Springer.

Levitt, B. E. (2005a). Non-directivity: The foundational attitude. In B. E. Levitt (Ed.), *Embracing non-directivity: Reassessing person-centered theory and practice in the 21st century* (pp. 5–16). Ross-on-Wye: PCCS Books.

Levitt, B. E. (2005b). *Embracing non-directivity: Reassessing person-centered theory and practice in the 21st century.* Ross-on-Wye: PCCS Books.

Linley, P. A., & Joseph, S. (Eds). (2004a). *Positive psychology in practice.* Hoboken, NJ: Wiley.

Linley, P. A., & Joseph, S. (2004b). Positive change following trauma and adversity: A review. *Journal of Traumatic Stress, 17,* 11–21.

Linley, P. A., Joseph, S., Cooper, R., Harris, S., & Meyer, C. (2003). Positive and negative changes following vicarious exposure to the September 11 terrorist attacks. *Journal of Traumatic Stress, 16,* 481–485.

Linley, P. A., Joseph, S., Harrington, S., & Wood, A. M. (2006). Positive psychology: Past, present, and (possible) future. *The Journal of Positive Psychology, 1,* 3–16.

Linley, P. A., Joseph, S., & Loumidis, K. (2005). Trauma work, sense of coherence, and positive and negative changes in therapists. *Psychotherapy and Psychosomatics, 74,* 185–188.

Littlewood, R., & Lipsedge, M. (1993). *Aliens and alienists: Ethnic minorities and psychiatry* (3rd ed.). London: Routledge.

Lopez, S. J., & Snyder, C. R. (Eds). (2003). *Positive psychological assessment: A handbook of models and measures.* Washington, DC: American Psychological Association.

Lopez, S. J., & Snyder, C. R. (2009). *Oxford handbook of positive psychology.* New York: Oxford University Press.

Lyons, J. A. (1991). Strategies for assessing the potential for positive adjustment following trauma. *Journal of Traumatic Stress, 4,* 93–111.

Lyubomirsky, S. (2008). The *how of happiness. A practical guide to getting the life you want.* London: Piatkus.

Ma, S. H., & Teasdale, J. D. (2004). Mindfulness-based cognitive therapy for depression: Replication and exploration of differential relapse prevention effects. *Journal of Consulting and Clinical Psychology, 72,* 31–40.

Maddux, J. E. (2002). Stopping the 'madness': Positive psychology and the deconstruction of the illness ideology and the DSM. In C. R. Snyder, & S. J. Lopez (Eds), *Handbook of positive psychology* (pp. 13–25). New York: Oxford University Press.

Maddux, J. E., Snyder, C. R., & Lopez, S. J. (2004). Toward a positive clinical psychology: Deconstructing the illness ideology and constructing an ideology of human strengths and potential. In P. A. Linley & S. Joseph (Eds), *Positive psychology in practice* (pp. 320–334). Hoboken, NJ: Wiley.

Maddux, J.E., & Lopez, S. J. (2015). Deconstructing the illness ideology and constructing an ideology of human strengths and potential in clinical psychology. In S. Joseph (Ed.), *Positive psychology in practice: Promoting human flourishing in work, health, education and everyday life* (2nd ed.) (pp. 411–427). Hoboken, NJ: Wiley.

Martin, D. J., Garske, J. P., & Davis, M. K. (2000). Relation of the therapeutic alliance with outcome and other variables: A meta-analytic review. *Journal of Consulting and Clinical Psychology, 68,* 438–450.

Martin, J. (2004). *Adversarial growth following cancer.* Doctor of Clinical Psychology thesis, University of Warwick.

Martin, J., Tolosa, I., & Joseph, S. (2004). Adversarial growth following cancer and support from health professionals. *Health Psychology Update, 13,* 11–17.

Marzillier, J. (2004). Psychotherapy: Is evidence the answer? Letters page. *The Psychologist, 17,* 625–626.

Maslow, A. H. (1954). *Motivation and personality.* New York: Harper.

Maslow, A. H. (1968). *Toward a psychology of being.* New York: Van Nostrand.

Maslow, A. H. (1970). *Motivation and personality* (2nd ed.). New York: Harper & Row.

Maslow, A. H. (1969). A theory of metamotivation: The biological rooting of the value-life. In A. J. Sutich and M. A. Vich (Eds), *Readings in humanistic psychology* (pp. 153–199). New York: Free Press.

Maslow, A. H. (1993). *The farther reaches of human nature*. New York: Penguin Arkana.

May, R. (1994). Contributions of existential psychotherapy. In R. May, E. Angel, & H. F.Ellenberger (Eds), *Existence* (pp. 37–91). Northvale, NJ: Jason Aronson. (Original work published 1958.)

McMillen, J. C., & Fisher, R. H. (1998). The perceived benefit scales: Measuring perceived positive life changes after negative events. *Social Work Research, 22*, 173–187.

Mearns, D. (2013). Foreword. In R. Know, D. Murphy, S. Wiggins, & M. Cooper, (Eds), *Relational depth: New perspectives and developments* (pp. vii-ix). Basingstoke: Palgrave.

Mearns, D., & Cooper, M. (2005). *Working at relational depth in counselling and psychotherapy*. London: Sage.

Mearns, D., Thorne, B., & McLeod, J. (2013). *Person-centred counselling in action* (4th ed.). London: Sage.

Merry, T. (1999). *Learning and being in person-centred counselling: A text book for discovering theory and developing practice*. Ross-on-Wye: PCCS Books.

Merry, T. (2004). Classical client-centred therapy. In P. Sanders, (2004). *The tribes of the person-centred nation: An introduction to the schools of therapy related to the person-centred approach* (pp. 21–44). Ross-on-Wye: PCCS Books:

Myers, D. G. (2004). Human connections and the good life: Balancing individuality and community in public policy. In P. A. Linley, & S. Joseph (Eds), *Positive psychology in practice* (pp. 641–657). Hoboken, NJ: Wiley.

Miller, W. R., & Rollnick, S. (2002). Motivational interviewing: Preparing people for change (2nd ed.). New York: Guilford Press.

Milne, D. (1999). Editorial: Important differences between the 'scientist-practitioner' and the 'evidence-based practitioner'. *Clinical Psychology Forum, 133*, 5–9.

Murphy, D., Duggan, M., & Joseph, S. (2013a). Relationship-based social work and its compatibility with the person-centred approach: Principled versus instrumental perspectives. *British Journal of Social Work, 43*, 703–719.

Murphy, D., & Joseph, S. (2013). Putting the relationship at the heart of trauma therapy. In D. Murphy & S. Joseph (Eds), *Trauma and the therapeutic relationship: Approaches to process and practice*. Houndmills: Palgrave Macmillan.

Murphy, D., & Joseph, S. (in press). Person-centered therapy: Past, present and future orientation. In D. A. Cain, K. Keenan, & S. Rubin (Eds), *Handbook of humanisitic psychotherapies*. Washington, DC: American Psychological Association.

Nafstad, H. (2015). Historical, philosophical, and epistemological perspectives. In S. Joseph (Ed.), *Positive psychology in practice: Promoting human flourishing in work, health, education and everyday life* (2nd ed.) (pp. 9–29). Hoboken, NJ: Wiley.

Neff, K.D. (2003). Self-compassion: An alternative conceptualization of a healthy attitude toward oneself. *Self and Identity, 2*, 85–101.

Neff, K. D., Kirkpatrick, K. L., & Rude, S. S. (2007). Self-compassion and adaptive psychological functioning. *Journal of Research in Personality, 41*, 139–154.

Neff, K. D., & Vonk, R. (2009). Self-compassion versus global self-esteem: Two different ways of relating to oneself. *Journal of Personality, 77*, 23–50.

Nelson-Jones, R. (1984). *Personal responsibility counselling and therapy: An integrative approach*. London: Harper & Row.

Niemiec, R. M. (2013). VIA character strengths: Research and practice (the first 10 years). In H. H. Knoop, & A. Delle Fave (Eds), *Well-being and cultures: Perspectives on positive psychology* (pp. 11–30). New York: Springer.

Norcross, J. C. (Ed.). (2001). Empirically supported therapy relationships: Summary of the Division 29 Task Force [Special Issue]. *Psychotherapy, 38*, 4.

Norem, J. K. (October, 2003). *Critiques and limitations of positive psychology*. Roundtable discussion at the second international positive psychology summit, Washington, DC.

O'Connell, B. (2005). *Solution-focused therapy* (2nd ed.). London: Sage.

O'Leary, V. E., & Ickovics, J. R. (1995). Resilience and thriving in response to challenge: An opportunity for a paradigm shift in women's health. *Women's health: Research on gender, behavior, and policy, 1*, 121–142.

Parks, A. C. (2004). Treating depressive symptoms with a positive intervention. Poster presented at 2004 international positive psychology summit, Sept 30–Oct 3.

Parks, A. C. (2015). Self-help interventions in positive psychology. In S. Joseph (Ed.), *Positive psychology in practice: Promoting human flourishing in work, health, education and everyday life* (2nd ed.) (pp. 237–248). Hoboken, NJ: Wiley.

Park, C. L. (1998). Stress-related growth and thriving through coping: The roles of personality and cognitive processes. *Journal of Social Issues, 54*, 267–277.

Park, C. L., Cohen, L. H., & Murch, R. (1996). Assessment and prediction of stress-related growth. *Journal of Personality, 64*, 71–105.

Patterson, T., & Joseph, S. (2006). Development of a self-report measure of unconditional positive self-regard. *Psychology and psychotherapy: Theory, research, and practice, 79*, 557–570.

Patterson, T. G., & Joseph, S. (2007a). Person-centered personality theory: Support from self-determination theory and positive psychology. *Journal of Humanistic Psychology, 47*, 117–139.

Patterson, T.G., & Joseph, S. (2007b). Outcome measurement in person-centered practice. In R. Worsley and S. Joseph (Eds), *Person-centered practice: Case studies in positive psychology* (pp. 200–217). Ross-on-Wye: PCCS Books.

Patterson, T. G., & Joseph, S. (2013). Unconditional positive self-regard: A person-centred approach to facilitating a non-contingent relationship with inner experiencing. In M. E. Bernard (Ed.), *The strength of self-acceptance: Theory, practice and research* (pp. 93–106). New York: Springer.

Pauwels, B. G. (2015). The uneasy – and necessary – role of the negative in positive psychology. In S. Joseph (Ed.), *Positive psychology in practice: Promoting human flourishing in work, health, education and everyday life* (2nd ed.) (pp. 807–821). Hoboken, NJ: Wiley.

Pavot, W., & Diener, E. (2004). Findings on subjective well-being: Applications to public policy, clinical interventions, and education. In P. A. Linley & S. Joseph (Eds), *Positive psychology in practice* (pp. 679–692). Hoboken, NJ: Wiley.

Payne, A., & Liebling-Kalifani, H., & Joseph, S. (2007). Client-centred group therapy for survivors of interpersonal trauma: A pilot investigation. *Counselling and Psychotherapy Research, 7*, 100–105.

Peterson, C. (2006). The values in action (VIA) classification of strengths. In M. Csikszentmihalyi, & I. Csikszentmihalyi (Eds), *A life worth living: Contributions to positive psychology* (pp. 29–48). New York, NY: Oxford University Press.

Peterson, C. (2007). *A primer in positive psychology*. New York: Oxford University Press.

Prati, G., & Pietrantoni, L. (2009). Optimism, social support, and coping strategies as factors contributing to posttraumatic growth: A meta-analysis. *Journal of Loss and Trauma, 14*, 364–388.

Proctor, G. (2005). Clinical psychology and the person-centred approach: An uncomfortable fit. In S. Joseph & R. Worsley (Eds), *Person-centred psychopathology: A positive psychology of mental health* (pp. 276–292). Ross-on-Wye: PCCS Books.

Proctor, G., Cooper, M., Sanders, P., & Malcolm, B. (Eds). (2006). *Politicizing the person-centred approach: An agenda for social change*. Ross-on-Wye: PCCS books.

Prouty, G. (1990). Pre-therapy: A theoretical evolution in the person-centred/experiential psychotherapy of schizophrenia and retardation. In G. Lietaer, J. Rombauts, & R. Van Balen (Eds), *Client-centred and experiential psychotherapy in the nineties* (pp. 645–658). Leuven: University of Leuven Press.

Rank, O. (1936). *Truth and reality: A life history of the human will*. New York: Knopf.

Rashid, T. (2015b). Strength-based assessment. In S. Joseph (Ed.), *Positive psychology in practice: Promoting human flourishing in work, health, education and everyday life* (2nd ed.) (pp. 519–542). Hoboken, NJ: Wiley.

Rashid, R. (2015b). Positive psychotherapy: A strength-based approach. *The Journal of Positive Psychology, 10*, 25–40.

Rathunde, K. (2001). Toward a psychology of optimal human functioning: What positive psychology can learn from the 'experiential turns' of James, Dewey, and Maslow. *Journal of Humanistic Psychology, 41*, 135–153.

Reeve, J., Nix, G., & Hamm, D. (2003). Testing models of the experience of self-determination in intrinsic motivation and the conundrum of choice. *Journal of Educational Psychology, 95*, 375–392.

Rennie, D. L. (1998). *Person-centred counselling: An experiential approach*. London: Sage.

Resnick, S., Warmoth, A., & Serlin, I. A. (2001). The humanistic psychology and positive psychology connection: Implications for psychotherapy. *Journal of Humanistic Psychology, 41*, 73–101.

Robbins, B. D. (2015). Building bridges between humanistic and positive psychology. In S. Joseph (Ed.), *Positive psychology in practice: Promoting human flourishing in work, health, education and everyday life* (2nd ed.) (pp. 31–45). Hoboken, NJ: Wiley.

Rogers, C. R. (1942). *Counseling and psychotherapy: Newer concepts in practice*. Boston: Houghton Mifflin.

Rogers, C. R. (1951). *Client-centred therapy: Its current practice, implications and theory*. Boston: Houghton Mifflin.

Rogers, C. R. (1957). The necessary and sufficient conditions of therapeutic personality change. *Journal of Consulting Psychology, 21*, 95–103.

Rogers, C. R. (1959). A theory of therapy, personality and interpersonal relationships, as developed in the client-centered framework. In S. Koch (Ed.), *Psychology: A study of a science, Vol. 3: Formulations of the person and the social context* (pp. 184–256). New York: McGraw Hill.

Rogers, C. R. (1961). *On becoming a person*. Boston: Houghton Mifflin.

Rogers, C. R. (1963a). The actualizing tendency in relation to 'motives' and to consciousness. In M. Jones (Ed.), *Nebraska symposium on motivation, Vol. 11* (pp. 1–24). Lincoln: University of Nebraska Press.

Rogers, C. R. (1963b). The concept of the fully functioning person. *Psychotherapy: Theory, research, and practice, 1*, 17–26.

Rogers, C. R. (1964). Toward a modern approach to values: The valuing process in the mature person. *Journal of Abnormal and Social Psychology, 68*, 160–167.

Rogers, C. R. (1969). *Freedom to learn.* Columbus, OH: Merrill.

Rogers, C. R. (1978). *Carl Rogers on personal power: Inner strength and its revolutionary impact.* London: Constable.

Rogers, C. R. (1980). *A way of being.* Boston: Houghton Mifflin.

Rollnick, S., & Miller, W. R. (1995). What is motivational interviewing? *Behavioural and Cognitive Psychotherapy, 23*, 325–334.

Rosenhan, D. L. (1973). On being sane in insane places. *Science, 179*, 250–258.

Rosenhan, D. L. (1975). The contextual nature of psychiatric diagnosis. *Journal of Abnormal Psychology, 84*, 442–452.

Roth, S., Lebowitz, L., & DeRosa, R. R. (1997). Thematic assessment of posttraumatic stress reactions. In J. P. Wilson, & T. M. Keane (Eds), *Assessing psychological trauma and PTSD* (pp. 512–528). New York: Guilford Press.

Ruini, C., & Fava, G. A. (2004). Clinical applications of well-being therapy. In P. A. Linley, & S. Joseph (Eds), *Positive psychology in practice* (pp. 371–387). Hoboken, NJ: Wiley.

Ruini, C., & Fava, G. A. (2015). Clinical applications of well-being therapy. In S. Joseph (Ed), *Positive psychology in practice: Promoting human flourishing in work, health, education, and everyday life* (2nd ed.) (pp. 463–487). Hoboken, NJ: Wiley.

Ryan, R. M. (1995). Psychological needs and the facilitation of integrative processes. *Journal of Personality, 63*, 397–427.

Ryan, R. M., & Deci, E. L. (2000). Self-determination theory and the facilitation of intrinsic motivation, social development, and well-being. *American Psychologist, 55*, 68–78.

Ryan, R. M., & Deci, E. L. (2001). On happiness and human potentials: A review of research on hedonic and eudaimonic well-being. *Annual Review of Psychology, 52*, 141–166.

Ryff, C. D. (1989). Happiness is everything, or is it? Explorations on the meaning of psychological well-being. *Journal of Personality and Social Psychology, 57*, 1069–1081.

Ryff, C. D., & Singer, B. H. (1996). Psychological well-being: Meaning, measurement, and implications for psychotherapy research. *Psychotherapy and Psychosomatics, 65*, 14–23.

Salovey, P., Caruso, D., & Mayer, J. D. (2004). Emotional intelligence in practice. In P. A. Linley, & S. Joseph (Eds), *Positive psychology in practice* (pp. 447–463). Hoboken, NJ: Wiley.

Salovey, P., Mayer, J. D., & Caruso, D. (2002). The positive psychology of emotional intelligence. In C. R. Snyder, & S. J. Lopez (Eds), *Handbook of positive psychology* (pp. 159–171). New York: Oxford University Press.

Sanders, P. (2004). The tribes of the person-centred nation: An introduction to the schools of therapy related to the person-centred approach. Ross-on-Wye: PCCS Books.

Sanders, P. (2005). Principled and strategic opposition to the medicalisation of distress and all of its apparatus. In S. Joseph, & R. Worsley (Eds), *Person-centred psychopathology: A positive psychology of mental health* (pp. 21–42). Ross-on-Wye: PCCS Books.

Sanders, P. (2013). The 'family' of person-centred and experiential therapies. In M. Cooper, P. F. Schmid, M. O'Hara, & A. C. Bohart (Eds). (2013). *The handbook of person-centred psychotherapy and counselling* (2nd ed.) (pp. 46–65). Basingstoke: Palgrave.

Sanders, P., & Hill, A. (2014). *Counselling for depression.* London: Sage.

Schmid, P. (2005). Facilitative responsiveness: Non-directiveness from anthropological, epistemological and ethical perspectives. In B. E. Levitt (Ed.), *Embracing nondirectivity: Reassessing person-centered theory and practice in the 21st century* (pp. 75–95). Ross-on-Wye: PCCS Books.

Schneider, K. J. (Ed.). (2008). *Existential-integrative psychotherapy: Guideposts to the core of practice*. New York: Routledge.

Schneider, K. (2011). Toward a humanistic positive psychology: Why can't we just get along? *Self and Society, 38*, 18–25.

Segal, Z. V., Williams, J. M. G., & Teasdale, J. D. (2002). *Mindfulness-based cognitive therapy for depression: A new approach to preventing relapse*. New York: Guildford Press.

Seligman, M. E. P. (1994). *What you can change and what you can't*. New York: Knopf.

Seligman, M. E. P. (1999). The president's address. *American Psychologist, 54*, 559–562.

Seligman, M. E. P. (2002). Positive psychology, positive prevention, and positive therapy. In C. R. Snyder, & S. J. Lopez (Eds), *Handbook of positive psychology* (pp. 3–9). New York: Oxford University Press.

Seligman, M. E. P. (2003a). Positive psychology: Fundamental assumptions. *The Psychologist, 16*, 126–127.

Seligman, M. E. P. (2003b). *Authentic happiness: Using the new positive psychology to realize your potential for lasting fulfilment*. New York: Free Press.

Seligman, M. E. P. (2004). Foreword. In P. A. Linley, & S. Joseph (Eds), *Positive psychology in practice* (pp. xi – xiii). Hoboken: Wiley.

Seligman, M. E. P (2004). *Character strengths and virtues: A handbook and classification*. Oxford: Oxford University Press.

Seligman, M. E. P., & Csikszentmihalyi, M. (2000). Positive psychology: An introduction. *American Psychologist, 55*, 5–14.

Seligman, M. E. P., & Peterson, C. (2003). Positive clinical psychology. In L. G. Aspinwall, & U. M. Staudinger (Eds), *A psychology of human strengths: Fundamental questions and future directions for a positive psychology* (pp. 305–317). Washington, DC: American Psychological Association.

Seligman, M. E. P., Rashid, T., & Parks, A. C. (2008). Positive psychotherapy. *American Psychologist, 61*, 774–788.

Seligman, M. E. P., Steen, T. A., Park, N., & Peterson, C. (2005). Positive psychology progress: Empirical validation of interventions. *American Psychologist, 60*, 410–421.

Shaw, A., Joseph, S., & Linley, P. A. (2005). Religion, spirituality and posttraumatic growth: A review. *Mental Health, Religion, and Culture, 8, 1–11*.

Sheldon, K. (2013). Self-determination theory, person-centered approaches, and personal goals: Exploring the links. In J. H. D. Cornelius-White, R. Motschnig-Pitrik, & M. Lux (Eds), *Interdisciplinary handbook of the person-centered approach: Research and theory* (pp. 227–244). New York: Springer.

Sheldon, K. M., Arndt, J., & Houser-Marko, L. (2003). In search of the organismic valuing process: The human tendency to move towards beneficial goal choices. *Journal of Personality, 71, 835–886*.

Sheldon, K. M., & Elliot, A. J. (1999). Goal striving, need satisfaction, and longitudinal well-being: The self-concordance model. *Journal of personality and social psychology, 76*, 482–497.

Sheldon, K. M., & Houser-Marko, L. (2001). Self-concordance, goal attainment, and the pursuit of happiness: Can there be an upward spiral? *Journal of Personality and Social Psychology, 80*, 152–165.

Sheldon, K. M., Joiner, T. E., Pettit, J. W., & Williams, G. (2003). Reconciling humanistic ideas and scientific clinical practice. *Clinical Psychology: Science and Practice, 10*, 302–315.

Sheldon, K. M., & Kasser, T. (2001). Goals, congruence, and positive well-being: New empirical support for humanistic theories. *Journal of Humanistic Psychology, 41*, 30–50.

Sheldon, K. M., & Kasser, T. (2001). Goals, congruence, and positive well-being: New empirical support for humanistic theories. *Journal of Humanistic Psychology, 41*, 30–50.

Sheldon, K. M., & King, L. (2001). Why positive psychology is necessary. *American Psychologist, 56*, 216–217.

Sheldon, K. M., & McGregor, H. A. (2000). Extrinsic value orientation and 'the tragedy of the commons'. *Journal of Personality, 68*, 383–411.

Shlien, J. M. (2003a). A criterion of psychological health. In P. Sanders (Ed.), *To lead an honourable life: Invitations to think about client-centered therapy and the person-centered approach* (pp. 15–18). Ross-on-Wye: PCCS Books.

Shlien, J. M. (2003b). Creativity and psychological health. In P. Sanders (Ed.), *To lead an honourable life: Invitations to think about client-centered therapy and the person-centered approach* (pp. 19–29). Ross-on-Wye: PCCS Books.

Sin, N. L., & Lyubomirsky, S. (2009). Enhancing well-being and alleviating depressive symptoms with positive psychology interventions: A practice friendly meta-analysis. *Journal of Clinical Psychology, 65*, 467–487.

Smail, D. (2005). *Power, interest and psychology: Elements of a social materialist understanding of distress*. Ross-on-Wye: PCCS books.

Smith, M. L., & Glass, G. V. (1977). Meta-analysis of psychotherapy outcome studies. *American Psychologist, 32*, 752–760.

Smith, M. L., Glass, G. V., & Miller, T. I. (1980). *The benefits of psychotherapy*. Baltimore: The Johns Hopkins University Press.

Snape, M. C. (1997). Reactions to a traumatic event: The good, the bad and the ugly? *Psychology, Health and Medicine, 2*, 237–242.

Snyder, C. R. (Ed.). (2000). *Handbook of hope: Theory, measures, and applications*. San Diego, CA: Academic Press.

Snyder, C. R., & Lopez, S. J. (Eds) (2002) *Handbook of positive psychology*. New York: Oxford University Press.

Snyder, C. R., & Lopez, S. J. (2007). *Positive psychology: The scientific and practical explorations of human strengths*. Thousand Oaks, CA: Sage.

Sternberg, R. J., & Grigorenko, E. L. (2001). Unified psychology. *American Psychologist, 56*, 1069–1079.

Stewart, I. (1989). *Transactional analysis counselling in action*. London: Sage.

Stiles, W. B., Barkham, M., Twigg, E., Mellor-Clark, J., & Cooper, M. (2006). Effectiveness of cognitive behavioural, person centred and psychodynamic therapies as practised in UK National Health Service settings. *Psychological Medicine, 36*, 555–566.

Sutich, A. J., & Vich, M. A. (1969). Introduction. In A. J. Sutich and M. A. Vich (Eds), *Readings in humanistic psychology* (pp. 1–18). New York: Free Press.

Tarragona, M. (2015). Positive psychology and life coaching. In S. Joseph (Ed.), *Positive psychology in practice: Promoting human flourishing in work, health, education and everyday life* (2nd ed.) (pp. 249–263). Hoboken, NJ: Wiley.

Taylor, E. (2001). Positive psychology and humanistic psychology: A reply to Seligman. *Journal of Humanistic Psychology, 41*, 13–29.

Taylor, S. E. (1983). Adjustment to threatening events: A theory of cognitive adaptation. *American Psychologist, 38*, 1161–1173.

Taylor, S. E., & Sherman, D. K. (2004). Positive psychology and health psychology: A fruitful liaison. In P. A. Linley, & S. Joseph (Eds), *Positive psychology in practice* (pp. 305–319). Hoboken, NJ: Wiley.

Teasdale, J. D., Moore, R. G., Hayhurst, H., Pope, M., Williams, S., & Segal, Z. V. (2002). Metacognitive awareness and prevention of relapse in depression: Empirical evidence. *Journal of Consulting and Clinical Psychology, 70*, 275–287.

Teasdale, J. D., Segal, Z. V., Williams, J. M. G., Ridgeway, V. A., Soulsby, J. M., & Lau, M. A. (2000). Prevention of relapse/recurrence in major depression by mindfulness-based cognitive therapy. *Journal of Consulting and Clinical Psychology, 68*, 615–623.

Tedeschi, R. G., & Calhoun, L. G. (1995). *Trauma and transformation: Growing in the aftermath of suffering.* Thousand Oaks, CA: Sage.

Tedeschi, R. G., & Calhoun, L. G. (1996). The posttraumatic growth inventory: Measuring the positive legacy of trauma. *Journal of Traumatic Stress, 9*, 455–471.

Tedeschi, R. G., & Calhoun, L. G. (2004). A clinical approach to posttraumatic growth. In P. A. Linley, & S. Joseph (Eds), *Positive psychology in practice* (pp. 405–419). Hoboken, NJ: Wiley.

Tedeschi, R. G., Calhoun, L. G., & Groleau, J. M. (2015). Clinical applications of posttraumatic growth. In S. Joseph (Ed.), *Positive psychology in practice: Promoting human flourishing in work, health, education, and everyday life* (2nd ed.) (pp. 503–518). Hoboken, NJ: Wiley.

Tedeschi, R. G., Park, C. L., & Calhoun, L. G. (Eds). (1998a). *Posttraumatic growth: Positive changes in the aftermath of crisis.* Mahwah, NJ: Lawrence Erlbaum.

Tedeschi, R. G., Park, C. L., & Calhoun, L. G. (1998b). Posttraumatic growth: Conceptual issues. In R. G.Tedeschi, C. L. Park, & L. G. Calhoun (Eds), *Posttraumatic growth: Positive changes in the aftermath of crisis.* Mahwah, NJ: Lawrence Erlbaum.

Thorne, B. (1992). *Carl Rogers.* London: Sage.

Traux, C. B., & Mitchell, K. M. (1971). Research on certain therapist interpersonal skills in relation to process and outcome. In A. E. Bergin and S. L. Garfield (Eds), *Handbook of psychotherapy and behavior change* (pp. 299–344). New York: Wiley.

Van Werde, D. (2005). Facing psychotic functioning: Person-centred contact work in residential psychiatric care. In S. Joseph, & R. Worsley (Eds), *Person-centred psychopathology: A positive psychology of mental health* (pp. 158–168). Ross-on-Wye: PCCS Books.

Veenhoven, R. (2004). Happiness as a public policy aim: The greatest happiness principle. In P. A. Linley, & S. Joseph (Eds), *Positive psychology in practice* (pp. 658–678). Hoboken, NJ: Wiley.

Vossler, A., Steffan, E., & Joseph, S. (2015). Counseling psychology and positive psychology: Towards a balanced integration. In S. Joseph (Ed), *Positive psychology in practice: Promoting human flourishing in work, health, education and everyday life* (2nd ed.) (pp. 429–441). Hoboken, NJ: Wiley.

Wampold, B. E. (2001). *The great psychotherapy debate: Models, methods, and findings.* Mahwah, NJ: Lawrence Erlbaum.

Ward, T., & Mann, R. (2004). Good lives and the rehabilitation of offenders: A positive approach to sex offender treatment. In P. A. Linley, & S. Joseph (Eds), *Positive psychology in practice* (pp. 598–616). Hoboken, NJ: Wiley.

Warner, M. (2002). Psychological contact, meaningful process and human nature. In G. Wyatt, & P. Sanders (Eds). *Rogers' therapeutic conditions, Vol. 4: Contact and perception* (pp. 76–95). Ross-on-Wye: PCCS Books.

Warner, M. (2005). A person-centered view of human nature, wellness, and psychopathology. In S. Joseph, & R. Worsley (Eds), *Person-centred psychopathology: A positive psychology of mental health* (pp. 91–109). Ross-on-Wye: PCCS Books.

Warner, M. (2008). *A client-centred approach to difficult client experiences.* Paper presented at the 5th congress of the world council of psychotherapy, Beijing, China.

Waterman, A. S. (1993). Two conceptions of happiness: Contrasts of personal expressiveness (eudaimonia) and hedonic enjoyment. *Journal of Personality and Social Psychology, 64,* 678–691.

Waterman, A. S. (2013). The humanistic psychology-positive psychology divide: Contrasts in philosophical foundations. *American Psychologist, 68,* 124–133.

White, R. W. (1959). Motivation reconsidered: The concept of competence. *Psychological Review, 66,* 297–333.

Wicks, R. J. (2008). *The resilient clinician.* New York: Oxford University Press.

Wilczynski, J., Brodley, B. T., & Brody, A. (2008). A rating system for studying nondirective client-centered interviews – revised. *The Person-Centered Journal, 15,* 34–57.

Wilkins, P. (2005a). Person-centred theory and 'mental illness'. In S. Joseph, & R. Worsley (Eds), *Person-centred psychopathology: A positive psychology of mental health* (pp. 43–59). Ross-on-Wye: PCCS Books.

Wilkins, P. (2005b). Assessment and 'diagnosis' in person-centred therapy. In S. Joseph, & R. Worsley (Eds), *Person-centred psychopathology: A positive psychology of mental health* (pp. 128–145). Ross-on-Wye: PCCS Books.

Williams, G. C., Cox, E. M., Hedberg, V. A., & Deci, E. L. (2000). Extrinsic life goals and health-risk behaviors among adolescents. *Journal of Applied Social Psychology, 30,* 1756–1771.

Wood, A.M, & Joseph, S. (2010) The absence of positive psychological (eudemonic) well-being as a risk factor for depression: A ten year cohort study. *Journal of Affective Disorders, 12,* 213–217

Wood, A. M., Linley, P. A., Maltby, J., Baliousis, M., & Joseph, S. (2008). The authentic personality: A theoretical and empirical conceptualization and the development of the authenticity scale. *Journal of Counselling Psychology, 55,* 385–399.

Worsley, R. (2009). *Process work in person-centred therapy* (2nd ed.). Basingstoke: Palgrave.

Worsley, R., & Joseph, S. (2007), (Ed.), *Person-centred practice: Case studies in positive psychology.* Ross-on-Wye: PCCS books.

Wyatt, G. (Ed.). (2001). *Rogers' therapeutic conditions: Evolution, theory and practice. Vol. 1: Congruence.* Ross-on-Wye: PCCS Books.

Wyatt, G., & Sanders, P. (Eds). (2001). *Rogers' therapeutic conditions: Evolution, theory and practice. Vol. 4: Contact and perception.* Ross-on-Wye: PCCS Books.

Yalom, I. (1980). *Existential therapy.* New York: Basic Books.

Yalom, I. (1989). *Love's executioner and other tales of psychotherapy.* London: Penguin Books.

Yalom, I. D. (2001). *The gift of therapy: Reflections on being a therapist.* London: Piatkus.

Index

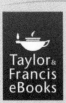